Getting the Most Out of Diabetes Camp

A Guide for Parents and Kids

American Diabetes Association®
Cure • Care • Commitment℠

Writer, Abe Ogden; *Director, Book Publishing,* John Fedor; *Associate Director, Consumer Books,* Sherrye Landrum; *Editor,* Mary Beth Keegan; *Production Manager,* Peggy M. Rote; *Composition,* Circle Graphics; *Cover Design,* Rikki Campbell; *Illustrator,* Jeff Johnston; *Printer,* Transcontinental Printing

Printed in Canada
1 3 5 7 9 10 8 6 4 2

The suggestions and information contained in this publication are generally consistent with the *Clinical Practice Recommendations* and other policies of the American Diabetes Association, but they do not represent the policy or position of the Association or any of its boards or committees. Reasonable steps have been taken to ensure the accuracy of the information presented. However, the American Diabetes Association cannot ensure the safety or efficacy of any product or service described in this publication. Individuals are advised to consult a physician or other appropriate health care professional before undertaking any diet or exercise program or taking any medication referred to in this publication. Professionals must use and apply their own professional judgment, experience, and training and should not rely solely on the information contained in this publication before prescribing any diet, exercise, or medication. The American Diabetes Association—its officers, directors, employees, volunteers, and members—assumes no responsibility or liability for personal or other injury, loss, or damage that may result from the suggestions or information in this publication.

∞ The paper in this publication meets the requirements of the ANSI Standard Z39.48-1992 (permanence of paper).

ADA titles may be purchased for business or promotional use or for special sales. For information, please write to Lee Romano Sequeira, Special Sales & Promotions, at the address below.

American Diabetes Association
1701 North Beauregard Street
Alexandria, Virginia 22311

Library of Congress Cataloging-in-Publication Data

Getting the most out of diabetes camp : a guide for parents and kids / American Diabetes Association

p. cm.

Includes index.

ISBN 1-58040-142-2 (pbk.)

1. Diabetes in children. 2. Diabetes in children—Patients—Care. 3. Camps for people with disabilities. I. American Diabetes Association.

RJ420.D5 G48 2002

618.92'462—dc21 2001056538

Contents

1

Why Diabetes Camp?

Summer camps have gotten a pretty bad rap the past few years. Maybe it's all those low-budget summer camp movies and predictable sitcom episodes, but most people associate summer camp with big bugs, bad food, and bored counselors. Then there are those camp directors who act like drill sergeants. No parent would put a kid through that, and no kid would want to have to go to such a place!

Especially when diabetes is involved.

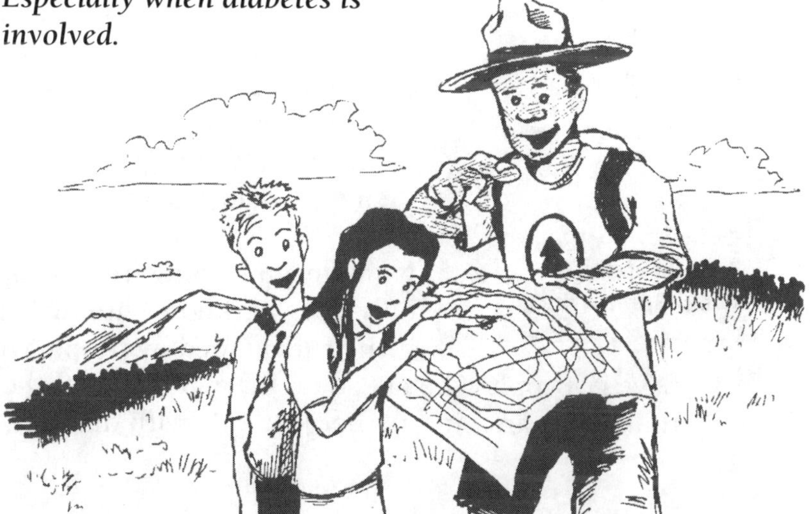

Luckily, camps are very different from the way they are depicted in movies. And this book should dispel any false notions you may have about camps for kids with diabetes, whether they are traditional (nondiabetes) camps or diabetes camps. Diabetes camps provide a great opportunity for children or teenagers who have diabetes to get to know others who have the condition, have fun, and learn something along the way. In fact, if you find the right camp, it can be an unforgettable adventure that your child will want to experience again and again. Just ask anyone who's already been there. Chances are, you'll get a glowing endorsement.

Suddenly, You're Not So Alone

"I had no idea there were this many kids with diabetes. I'm the only one in my school and I just figured it was that way all over. But there's lots of us out there and we all get together at camp."

Camper, Age 10, ADA Camp at Camp Green Lane

As you know, kids with diabetes are in the minority. This is especially true in small communities, where they may be the only ones in their school with the condition. You don't need a doctorate in psychology to know that this can have a pretty big impact on how a kid perceives herself and the world around her. Nobody wants to be an outsider; nobody wants to be excluded or different from the group. Unfortunately, this is how many children with diabetes feel.

Now, imagine going from being the only one you know with diabetes to being surrounded by people who have it, people who are going through many of the same things you are. And it's not just kids with diabetes, but also adult staff members, many of whom have had it for years and have gone on to live full, rich lives. You get to meet counselors who went through many of the things you are going through now and can share ways to cope with the problems and pitfalls of having diabetes. Suddenly you're not alone; you have someone you can identify with, someone who can help. This is how kids feel at diabetes camp. In fact, a family doctor or diabetes-care team member will often recommend diabetes camp for a child who is having a hard time dealing with his diabetes.

Safety at Camp

Kids with diabetes, and their parents, have a pretty extensive list of health and safety concerns. From nutrition to proper medical supplies to something as basic as staying properly hydrated, the list of things to be aware of can go on and on.

Over the years, due in part to the work of the American Diabetes Association (ADA) and other nonprofit organizations, traditional summer camps have come a long way in their ability to accommodate campers with different health needs. These traditional camps may not be as knowledgeable about diabetes as a camp specifically designed for kids with diabetes, but many kids with diabetes have had safe, wonderful times at these camps, so either camp can work for you, depending on your situation. (*See chapter 8 if you would like to know more about traditional camps for kids with diabetes.*)

At diabetes camps, many of the counselors have diabetes themselves, and if they don't, they have been thoroughly trained to handle any emergency that may arise. Furthermore, by keeping a close watch on things like meal plans,

glucose testing, and exercise, camps try to prevent such emergencies from happening in the first place.
Some of the safety features you should find at a diabetes camp include:

- well-trained and knowledgeable staff, usually made up of counselors who have diabetes
- on-site medical team
- medical facilities and supplies
- tailored nutrition information and guidance
- closely monitored and administered glucose testing, insulin injection, and pump maintenance
- activities that accommodate the needs and concerns of someone with diabetes
- overall focus on safety

For Kids Only:
The Best Thing about Camp

Ask any camper or counselor what their favorite thing about diabetes camp is, and they'll probably tell you it's being around other campers and counselors with diabetes. Sometimes you have so much in common with them and like them so much that you become friends for life.

But aside from making great friends, being around others who have diabetes can help you feel less alone. You start feeling a little better about yourself and your situation. Plus, you might even learn a few things, so you feel more confident. But not just from sitting in a classroom—in fact, most counselors agree that kids usually learn more about diabetes from hanging around and talking with other campers and the counselors than they do from any organized classes.

Camp Can Be Educational, Too

It's almost guaranteed that campers are going to come away from camp knowing something about diabetes that they didn't know before. While some camps do make classes part of the schedule, campers often learn more on their own than from the formal lessons. Kids will pick up a lot from friends, staff, and the classes, but education is usually not the primary focus of camp. Often the process just seems to happen on its own—when kids are talking quietly in the cabin bunks before bed, when campers or counselors are sitting around telling stories, or when campers learn from watching how others take care of themselves.

With this in mind, parents should realize that a camper isn't going to return from a one- or two-week overnight camp completely ready to take care of himself. Self-care takes time to master, and kids will learn it at the age and the pace that is right for them. Some kids start giving themselves insulin when they're six years old. Others don't even start their own testing until they're in their teens. Every child is different. However, most camps do teach various aspects of self-care, and many kids leave camp more self-sufficient than they were before.

But just because your child knows how to take care of himself, that doesn't necessarily mean he's itching to try it. Eventually, when he feels ready, your child will be ready to take on more responsibility for his own care. And this is probably where camp can be most influential. Whether or not your camper comes back with solid knowledge, it's a pretty safe bet he'll return with more self-confidence and a willingness to accept more responsibility for himself. This is the biggest step towards self-care.

Luckily for the kids, diabetes camp is not a clinic in the woods or an intensive seminar designed to produce completely independent kids who are ready and willing to handle their diabetes care. Yes, kids are going to learn something—probably quite a bit. But this shouldn't be the sole reason they're headed to camp (and it's certainly not the reason they want to go to camp). Diabetes camp is a place for kids with diabetes to get together with each other in a safe environment and have fun. If they happen to learn something along the way, great!

Dr. Richard Guthrie— I've Seen Lives Turned Around

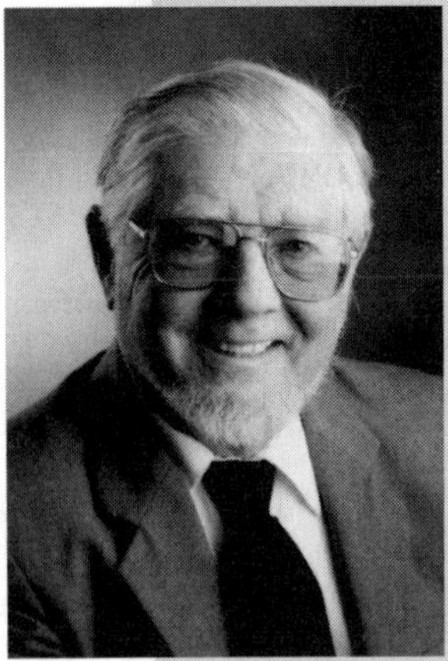

Dr. Richard Guthrie, along with his colleague, Dr. Don Etzwiler, has played an integral role in the development of diabetes camps across the United States. Since the early '70s, when diabetes camps were rare, Dr. Guthrie has not only worked to raise money for camps and improve standards, he and his wife have also run camps of their own. During this time, in which diabetes camps have grown to number more than 100 in North America alone, Guthrie has seen a lot of improvements in the camps. He has seen lives transformed as well.

"I can't begin to say how many lives I've seen turned around by diabetes camp. Hundreds—too many to count.

There's one kid I remember in particular, and his story is like those of a lot of kids I've known. When he first got to camp, he was out of control. He didn't want to take care of himself, so he didn't. He was headed down the wrong path. He didn't participate in any activities or follow any of the camp rules. He was very angry—angry that he had diabetes, that he had to suffer through this. He had the same question that a lot of kids with diabetes have, 'Why me?' And it made him very bitter.

"We worked with him all through the week, trying to get him to participate. By the end of camp, he was just starting to come around, but we didn't expect to see him back the next year. Well, to our surprise, he was one of the first kids to sign up for camp the next summer. When he came back, he wasn't completely transformed, but he was a lot more willing to participate and a little less self-destructive. And he came back every year, every summer he was there.

"Now he's a successful adult with a great career and a wonderful family, and we talk on a pretty regular basis. It's like he's one of my own kids—I feel so proud of him! And this isn't an isolated case—I've seen it countless times.

(*continued*)

> "You don't really think a summer camp could have such a profound effect on people, but it can. Just being with kids and other adults who have had similar experiences, people you can identify with, can really have a meaningful impact on your life. I know; I've seen it happen for the past 30 years."

Fun—The Most Important Reason of All

Safety, education, and boosted self-esteem are all good reasons to attend a diabetes camp, but the main reason to go to this or any other type of camp is simply to have fun. If you're having fun, all the other things will fall in line. You'll learn more, you'll be more willing to try new things, and you'll want to keep coming back year after year. Diabetes camping professionals say that if you really want to learn and use diabetes management skills, it will take several years of camp. Who would want to do something for that long that they disliked?

So what kind of fun stuff happens at diabetes camp? Well, that depends on the camp, which is why you need to do some research before writing a check and packing the kids' bags. At most camps you'll find a variety of activities. Some offer horseback riding, others might stress hiking and the outdoors. Some are centered on swimming, sports, or a specific interest, while others offer more general activities, leaving plenty of time for kids to get together, hang out, and make friends. Every camp is different, but one thing remains the same—they're all focused on giving campers a good time.

✦ ✦ ✦

These are just a few of the reasons why diabetes camp is an excellent choice for just about any kid with this condition. But chances are, you still have questions. How do you pick the right camp? How do you apply? What do you need once you're accepted? What accommodations do you need to make if you decide to send your child to a traditional camp? These are all things we'll discuss later in the book. But first, there's something more important that you need to decide: Is your child ready for camp?

2

Is Your Child Ready for Camp?

The camp brochures show kids riding horses, swimming, and singing around a campfire, and everyone looks like they're having a wonderful time. And it's true that a kid can have one of the best times of her life at camp, as long as she's ready. But some parents may not realize that if a child isn't ready, she can have a tough time. If your child has never stayed the night with a friend or gone to stay with a relative, she may not be ready for two weeks away from home. At this stage in her life, camp can turn from a fun-filled adventure into a frightening experience pretty quickly. And if your camper's first time at camp is traumatic, there's a chance she'll never want to go back.

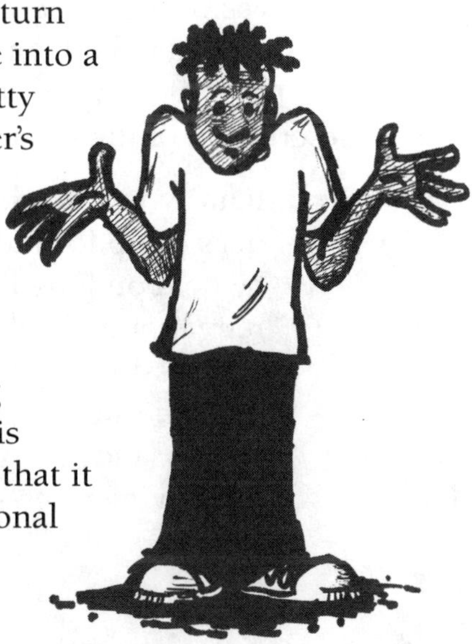

When it comes to deciding whether or not your child is ready for camp, remember that it has more to do with emotional maturity than it does with her ability to take care of herself. Any well-equipped camp will be prepared to handle all aspects of a child's diabetes care, from administering insulin and other medications to checking blood sugars and providing proper meals and nutritional guidance. Your child will be well taken care of. However, whether or not your child will be able to handle the emotional aspects of being away from home and interacting with other campers is another question altogether.

So how do you know when he *is* ready? It's a tough question, since each child's situation is unique. There are no definite rules about when your child is ready for camp, but there are signs you can look for to gauge how ready he is.

Types of Camps

Another consideration is the type of camp. Different camps are aimed at different age and maturity levels. Your camper may not be ready for a three-week sleepover camp two states away, but he might be just the right age for a week-long day camp. We'll discuss the types of camps in detail and what each has to offer in the next chapter, "Selecting the Best Camp." For now, here's a brief description of the three types.

- **Family weekend.** A family weekend is like a beginner's camp for kids with diabetes. These camps may be held on long holiday weekends, sometimes at a retreat or a nice hotel. The entire family is together, and sessions away from the parents are optional, so even the shyest kid can participate. It's a fun, safe way for kids to meet other kids with diabetes without having to be separated from parents.

- **Day camp.** Day camp is great for the younger camper who can handle spending a day away from parents, but isn't quite ready for overnight camp. Many day camps focus on kids aged four to eight, but they're also good for older kids. Usually running for about a week, they focus on low-intensity activities like crafts and other activities, swimming, and basic diabetes education.
- **Resident camp.** This is what most people think of as camp. At these overnight camps, kids sleep in bunks, usually in cabins. They stay at the camp (except for field trips) for the whole period, getting completely immersed in the camping experience. Of course, there's also a greater chance that they'll feel homesick. Ages vary, but if a child has been in school for a couple of years and has spent a long weekend with friends or family, he's probably mature enough for a resident camp. Some campers don't attend resident camps until they're eight or nine, but

A Note on Insulin Pumps

Insulin pumps are a recent and welcome addition to diabetes management and can be accommodated at camp. Planning and preparation are the key to success at camp with the pump. For example, it is not wise to begin insulin pump therapy within 6 to 8 weeks before camp. Pump therapy requires constant attention and calibration before the proper settings are achieved. During this period of adjustment, blood glucose can sometimes swing widely and uncontrollably. It could be risky if this happens at camp, when children are already experiencing the blood glucose fluctuations associated with increased activity and excitement. Camp can, however, be a good opportunity for children

(*continued*)

and families considering pump therapy to learn more about the pros and cons from fellow campers and staff.

Currently there are several different insulin pumps on the market. Typically 25–50% of campers are now on the pump when they come to camp. This creates unique challenges in the management of insulin delivery and impacts some program areas (for instance, adequate, dry, and labeled storage areas for pumps and set change supplies must be provided at pool and waterfront areas). In order to meet the needs of the child on a pump the camp staff must know the following:

- The brand of pump and supplies needed for operation
- The pump management routine used at home
- The child's level of confidence using the pump and changing sets

other children, such as one who has been in full-time day care, might be ready at a younger age.

The Good, the Bad, and the Buggy

One of the best ways to determine whether or not your child is ready for camp is to sit down and talk with her. Go over all the different aspects of camping; try to show her the whole picture. If she envisions a week of blissful horse rides through the mountains and gourmet dinners, she may be terribly disappointed with the bugs and rustic cabins. Of course, you don't want to scare her with a completely negative picture—camp can be lots of fun. Here are some things you might discuss:

- Getting along with staff and other campers
- Following camp rules and schedules

- Feeling strange in an unfamiliar place
- Being separated from family and friends (and having the chance to make new friends!)
- Learning new skills, such as archery, canoeing, and horseback riding
- Having fun!

If she still has serious reservations about overnight camps once she knows what's involved, you might want to check out day-camp options first. There will be more opportunities to go to overnight camp in the future, and sometimes it's best to take it slowly, one step at a time. If, on the other hand, it looks like she is comfortable with the idea, you're probably ready to go.

While it's true that many kids who didn't really want to go to camp end up having a great time and come back year after year, camp shouldn't be something that's forced on them. It might take a little coaxing and persuading, but she'll be more receptive to the idea if she makes the final decision herself. At very least, parents and child should discuss it together, as a family.

> "When I first came to camp, I was scared to wake up the counselors when I had a problem at night. But this is important and I finally learned that they wouldn't get mad."
>
> **Camper, Age 9, ADA Camp at Camp Green Lane**

Get Feedback from Others

Another good way to tell whether a camper is ready is by talking to others who know your situation and your son or daughter. Talk with members of your diabetes-care team or your family doctor. They can usually offer sound advice and possibly, some recommendations of good camps.

Other families who have sent children to diabetes camp are another great resource. They know first-hand the pleasures and pitfalls and can share their experiences. If you don't know anyone else with type 1 diabetes, the American Diabetes Association's monthly magazine, *Diabetes Forecast*, has a section devoted to contacting others, "Making Friends." You could also contact your ADA regional office to find others who have attended camp and would be willing to discuss what they know. (For legal reasons, the American Diabetes Association does not provide a forum for contacting children with diabetes.)

> "It's hard to tell when a kid is ready for camp. It really depends on the kid. I would say that the staff plays a pretty big role. The right counselor can help any kid have a good time—there's really no age limit. I've seen five-year-olds at camp, although for some kids, that might be a little young for an overnight camp. But with good people who know what they're doing, any kid's going to have fun."
>
> **Mike, Counselor, Kansas City ADA Diabetes Camp at Camp Shawnee**

But Are You Ready for Your Child to Go to Camp?

This is the one question most parents aren't prepared for. In the process of choosing camps and making sure your child has everything he or she needs, parents sometimes lose sight of the fact that they're also going to be separated from their kids. Because children with diabetes have always needed extra attention and care, much more than a child without diabetes would, many parents eventually get a little overprotective. This is normal. When it comes to something that takes the health of your child out of your hands, any caring parent is going to be diligent.

So the thing to ask yourself is, are you really ready to let your child leave for an extended period of time? Can you let qualified professionals take responsibility for her? If you've thoroughly researched the camp, you know that it can handle any medical emergency that might come up. Are *you* emotionally ready to make that leap?

You are probably going to miss your child while she's gone, but the thing to keep in mind is that she is headed to a safe and controlled environment and is in the hands of people who know what they're doing. In fact, your child is probably safer at camp than anywhere else. And remember that she'll be back home soon. Being away from a child can be emotional for any parent, and it's natural to worry. Just try to make sure your worrying doesn't interfere with a potentially good time for your child. And for yourself.

Every parent needs a break once in awhile, some time for yourself or to be with your spouse, away from the duties of being a parent. Having a kid with diabetes can be especially difficult for parents, since they are responsible for the child's daily health regimen. So camp can be a good way to get some time for yourselves. In fact, summer camp can be a little bit of a vacation for parents, too.

You Won't Know 'Til You Try It

The truth is, no matter how much you discuss it, research it, or venture a guess, you'll never know whether or not your child is ready for camp until he or she has actually gone. Sometimes, an enthusiastic camper finds that being away from his parents is harder than he thought. (*For more on this subject, see chapter 7, "Homesickness."*) On the other hand, kids that were a little leery can find that camp is so exciting and fun that they don't miss home nearly as much as they thought they would. You just never know.

We can all get a little scared by new things and new situations. It's human nature. In the right hands, any kid is ready for the adventures of camp life. This is why a competent and caring staff is so important. A good counselor can help a camper who is nervous get over his fears and really take advantage of all the camp has to offer.

So how do you know if the staff is up to the task ahead? We'll discuss that in the next chapter. Just keep in mind that when it comes to choosing a camp, the staff is probably the most important factor to consider.

3

Selecting the Best Camp

We've talked about the advantages of diabetes camp and how to assess whether or not your child is ready for camp. Now comes one of the more difficult decisions—selecting the best camp. Every family is different, so personal taste, practical concerns, and a little bit of intuition are key factors in your decision. We can't tell you which camp is right for you—that's your choice. We can, however, tell you what to expect from different kinds of camps and some of the characteristics of a well-run camp. After that, it's up to you.

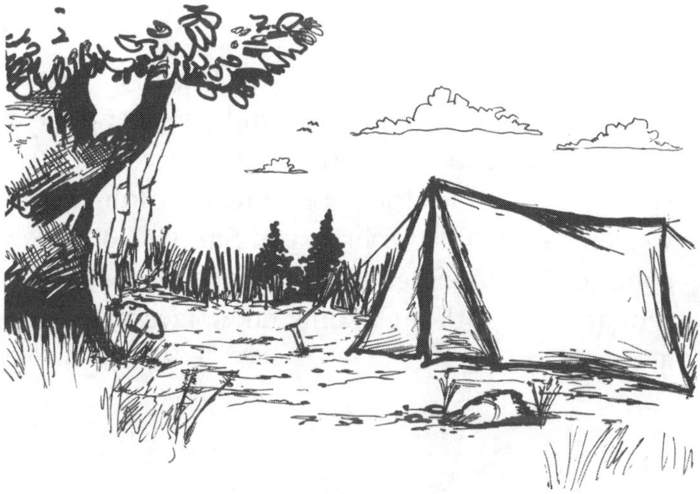

When should you start looking for a camp? Right now! It's never too early to start looking into camps. If you want a camp for this summer, it's best to start looking by February. The earlier you get started, the better chance you have of getting into the camp you want. Also, camp dates are often limited to one or two weeks in the summer, so you may need to plan your other summer activities around their schedule.

Which Type of Camp Is Right for You?

The first decision you need to make when selecting a camp is which type of camp you want. We talked briefly in the last chapter about the types of camps that are best for different age groups and mindsets. Now, we'll get a little more in-depth and see what each type has to offer.

The family weekend

Technically, family weekends aren't exactly camps. They take less time, don't require separation from parents, and may not be held in a camp setting. Family weekends bring kids with diabetes and their parents together with other families to share stories, gather information, and just have a good time.

But family weekends aren't just a bunch of people sitting around and talking. A good family weekend has planned activities, diabetes education, and a vacation atmosphere. Sometimes they're planned for long holiday weekends, often from Friday to Sunday, to give everyone enough time together. They're typically held at hotels or retreat centers, though some take place in a campground atmosphere.

Of all the camps available, family weekends are probably the most varied. No two are alike. They are usually less structured than traditional camps and are typically organized with the help of local parents. Attending a family weekend also doesn't require much research, since the kids will be with a parent most of the time and considerations such as facilities, safety record, and staff aren't important. A family weekend is probably the best choice if:

- the camper isn't quite ready for a traditional camp
- the parent wants to be more actively involved
- your family mainly wants to meet other kids with diabetes and their parents

Family weekends aren't listed on the ADA list of camps in the resource section of this book, so for the most up-to-date listings, please visit *www.diabetes.org/wizdom/liveitup/camp.shtml*. To find out if there are any family weekends scheduled for your area or to help organize a family weekend, call 1-888-DIABETES (342-2383) to find out the number for your American Diabetes Association regional office. They should be able to provide you with any information you need.

The day camp

Day camps are a great way for kids with diabetes to begin their camp experience. Day camps are much more involved than family weekends, are normally situated in a more nature-rich environment (if not a campground, then a ranch, park, or recreation center), and include many of the activities of a resident camp. Since campers go home at the end of each day, they're not as stressful as overnight camps, but they still allow for some traditional camp fun. In addition, day camps may be better for working parents, since the camps provide adult supervision during the day and may last longer than overnight camps.

Many campers, especially younger ones, start off by attending a day camp. Day camps allow for socializing with other campers, and they incorporate education, but usually at an easier pace than at resident camps. This allows the children to move at their own pace until they feel comfortable enough to take on more. And they almost always do want something more. If a kid has a good time at day camp, resident camp usually follows, and the transition is easier.

Some of the things a camper will usually find at a day camp include:

- a nature-oriented environment
- group activities, such as swimming, hiking, and scavenger hunts
- crafts
- low-level educational activities
- lots of other kids, counselors, and staff with diabetes
- a great experience!

In contrast to family weekends, day camps inherently bring with them more concerns. Since parents won't be around all day, it's important to have inspected the facilities, met the staff, and ensured that supervision and medical facilities are adequate. If it's an ADA-run camp, you probably won't find any problems. But it's always good to meet the staff and inspect the grounds, even if it's only for peace of mind.

The great thing about day camp is that any kid can enjoy what it has to offer. Since you don't stay the night, younger kids aren't intimidated, and with all of the activities provided, older kids enjoy it, too. In fact, some kids go to day camp well into their teens, especially if there isn't a resident camp nearby.

Day camp is probably the best option for you if:

- the camper isn't quite ready for a week or two away from his parents but wants a more camplike experience than a family weekend can offer
- your child wants to meet other kids and adults with diabetes
- there aren't any resident camps in the area

The resident camp

When you started thinking about summer camp, this is probably the type of camp you had in mind. In fact, a lot of people are surprised to learn there are other types of camp. But as you've seen, a resident camp is just one type of camp available to kids with diabetes. Some people claim, however, that they're the most fun.

Resident camps vary widely. Some run for three or four days at local college campuses; others for weeks in remote areas of the country. Some provide a summer retreat for hundreds of diabetes campers; others are much smaller. A few focus on certain sports or activities, while others just provide a natural environment and a variety of activities.

Most diabetes camps can be found close to home (or at least within the state), run for about a week, and accept about 40 to 60 campers. Many nondiabetes campgrounds set aside one or two weeks each summer to hold diabetes camp, but others are exclusively diabetes camps, holding continuous sessions all season long.

Diabetes camp is considered a specialty camp, and it's hard to locate a camp that focuses on two "specialties" at the same time, such as diabetes and basketball. Usually, diabetes camps just focus on a variety of regular summer camp activities. Each camp is different, but you'll probably find some combination of the following activities:

- Swimming
- Boating and canoeing
- Sports—softball, basketball, and soccer, for example
- Hiking
- Horseback riding
- Archery
- Crafts
- Campfire gatherings
- Team exercises, such as a ropes course
- Diabetes education

Basically, you'll find everything you've come to expect from a regular summer camp, plus more! And these are just the scheduled activities. The real fun is hanging out with other kids who have diabetes and making friends.

Of course, resident camps bring more concerns than the other types of diabetes camps. Since the campers stay for extended periods of time, you need to make sure that the camp is in good shape and that you're familiar with the staff. You should request a brochure or other promotional information, but they're not going to reveal anything negative in the brochure, so you should go to the campground yourself and see what it's really like. It's up to you to see what's really happening at the camp.

> "I went to a day camp for a couple of years and it was fun. But I learned a lot more at resident camp."
>
> **Camper, Age 14, Camp Nejeda**

Ask any counselor at a resident camp what the biggest problem is, and they'll all tell you the same thing—homesickness. Before heading off to resident camp, make sure your camper is ready for what lies ahead. Rest assured that being homesick is a natural reaction and that as the week goes along, it will get better. Of course, having a child away from home can be difficult for you as well as your child, so be prepared for a touch of "empty nest syndrome" yourself!

Getting Information on Camps

After you've decided on what type of camp best suits your needs, it's time to start gathering information on camps in your area. There are thousands of summer camps across the nation, but only a portion of those offer diabetes camps. Sifting through all the camps across the country can be a daunting task, so limiting your options to those in your area is a good place to start.

One of the best ways to get information on a diabetes camp is to contact your regional ADA office. Call 1-888-DIABETES to get in touch with the nearest one, or you can visit *www.diabetes.org/wizdom/ liveitup/camps.shtml/* and check

For Kids Only: What Kind of Camp Do You Want?

A family weekend is probably right for you if:

- You aren't quite ready for a traditional camp
- Your father or mother wants to be more actively involved
- You are most interested in meeting others with diabetes

Day camp is probably the best choice if you:

- aren't quite ready for a week or two away from your parents
- want more of the camp experience than a family weekend offers
- want to meet other kids and adults with diabetes
- don't have any resident camps nearby
- want to have fun all day

Resident camp is probably the best choice if you:

- are ready for a week or two away from home
- want a complete camping experience
- hope to meet other kids and adults with diabetes
- want to have loads of fun, day and night

the list of camps to see which ones are closest to you and when they are being held. A few camps run continuous sessions throughout the summer, but many others only run them for one or two weeks a year. So, as we said before, you should start looking as early as possible.

Your local ADA office will probably have pamphlets and brochures for the camps in your area, but it might be necessary to contact the camp directly for more information, especially if it isn't exclusively a diabetes camp. The person in charge of camps at the ADA office can tell you how to get in touch with the camp you're interested in. But be prepared. One you start contacting camps directly you can expect a mountain of promotional materials coming your way—from videos to pamphlets to book-length brochures. While these items can be a big help, remember that they try to present the camp in the best possible light. They are no substitute for visiting a camp and doing outside research of your own.

What to Look For in a Camp

You've decided what type of camp you're interested in and contacted your local American Diabetes Association office. You've got loads of promotional materials either headed your way or piled in front of you. Now what? Do you pick your camp based on the best-looking brochure? The one whose kids look happiest in the pictures? The camp that looks best?

Basically, there are seven key elements you should check in order to select the best camp:

- Staff
- Location
- Cost
- Size
- Facilities
- Accreditation
- Safety record

Staff

Never underestimate the importance of the staff. These are the people who will be looking after your child while

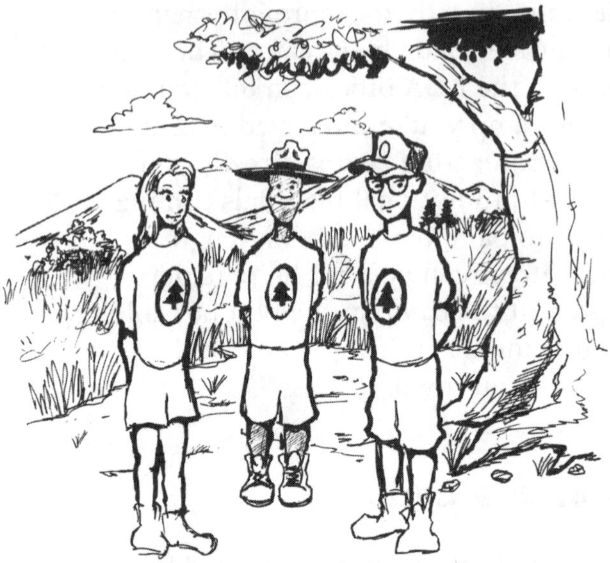

he's at camp. This is a big responsibility at all camps, but it's even more important when the camper has diabetes. Since many diabetes camp counselors are college students or volunteers, it may not be possible to meet them while you're visiting camps in the off-season. However, when researching staff requirements, make sure that:

- there is a good medical-staff-to-camper ratio (1:10 is just about right)
- the camp recruits staff who have diabetes themselves
- the counselors who don't have diabetes have had at least five to seven hours of training in diabetes care
- some of the counselors have attended or have previous experience with diabetes camp
- the camp hires counselors who are warm, friendly, and good with kids

Keep in mind that the safety of our campers is the first priority of the American Diabetes Association. As a child care provider, ADA complies with all state and federal laws as well as American Camping Association (ACA) standards, including the background search of all staff, the verification of medical licenses, and mandatory reporting of suspected child abuse and neglect.

You'll probably have the opportunity to speak with the camp director, who can give you a basic rundown of the staff. Once camp season starts, try to visit and meet with the staff, even if you've already committed to the camp. Talking with the friendly and dedicated people who will be guiding and supervising your camper can make everyone involved feel more at ease.

Location

Location can be a big concern when it comes to diabetes camps. Not all regions of the country offer diabetes camp, especially less populated areas. Some campers may have to travel pretty far from home to find a diabetes camp. If you're worried about your child feeling homesick, this extra distance can be both a detriment and a benefit. Obviously, the thought of being so far away from your family can make the homesickness much worse. But sometimes, when parents can't just come and pick a child up from camp, a camper is forced to cope with the situation much better, since leaving isn't really an option. If a camper is going to a distant camp, it would be ideal to have some family nearby, just in case.

Often, the camp that's nearest to you is the best option, depending on the type of camp and the environment you're looking for. If a camper has already been to the same camp a couple of times, he might want to try somewhere new for a change. If you live on the coast, he might want to visit a camp in the mountains. If you live in the Midwest, he might want to go to a camp near the ocean. Or he might just want to stay right where he is.

A Note on Picking Up Your Child at the End of Camp

If you plan to have someone other than a parent pick up your child at the end of the camp session, it is imperative that the camp staff know ahead of time. It is against ADA regulations (and should be against any camp's regulations) to release a child to an unauthorized person, for obvious safety reasons. So if you plan on having another family member or friend pick up your camper from camp, be sure to let the camp staff know well ahead of time in writing.

Cost

The American Diabetes Association prides itself on offering quality camps at a competitive rate. Our wish is to make cost the least of your concerns when it comes to selecting a camp. If cost is a consideration, many diabetes camps offer some type of scholarship based on family income. A few are subsidized by local service organizations and are free. No nationwide scholarship program exists right now, but if you feel you need financial assistance, speak with your local ADA office and the director of the camp you're interested in. They will be able to provide more information on what scholarships and financial aid programs are available.

If you don't qualify for financial assistance, remember that diabetes camp is an investment in your child's happiness and health, so whatever the cost, it's almost certainly worth it. (If you would like to donate money so that others can attend diabetes camp, talk with someone at your ADA office.)

Size

Camps vary dramatically in size, from programs with 15 campers to those with hundreds of campers. The camp size that's right for your child depends on the experience you're looking for.

Smaller camps offer more intimacy among campers and counselors and may provide for closer supervision and more direct guidance from those in charge. It also makes it easier to conduct certain activities, like hiking and camping, that would be impossible with a large group. However, since smaller camps generate less money than larger camps, they can either be more expensive or less equipped.

On the other hand, larger camps provide a chance to meet lots of other kids with diabetes from a variety of different backgrounds. They're occasionally less expensive and offer more expansive facilities. With greater numbers of kids, it's easier to play organized sports, such as softball and soccer.

Facilities

This is where promotional materials for camps can be the most misleading. Brochures often show picturesque facilities perched atop breathtaking landscapes with lakes and volleyball courts and horses and kids glowing with blissful expressions painted across their faces. While most camps are far from dilapidated, they usually aren't as idyllic as their promotional materials make them out to be. Before committing to any camp, it's always best to inspect the grounds yourself, if only to lessen the shock between marketing and reality. Keep in mind that if you visit a camp during the off-season, there's probably going to be some renovation and landscaping being done, and it won't look nearly as good as when camp starts. Still, you can check structures like bunks, bathrooms, and dining areas for any major problems.

If the ADA runs the camp you're looking into, everything should be up to speed and completely safe for your camper. The ADA requires that all camps meet high standards for safety, cleanliness, and structural soundness. If the ADA doesn't run the camp, there's no real guarantee, unless it's accredited by the American Camping Association (ACA). No matter what, it's always best to see the campground for yourself.

Accreditation

One of the first things you need to look for in a camp is accreditation from the ACA. The ACA is a national organization dedicated to providing the utmost in camping quality. It is the only nationally recognized body that accredits all types of camps throughout the United States. If a camp has received ACA accreditation, it has demonstrated that it meets stringent standards of health, safety, and program quality. For more information on the American Camping Association and its requirements for accreditation, visit *www.acacamps.org*.

All camps run by the American Diabetes Association are required to meet ACA standards for accreditation. However, some camps, usually day camps, don't meet certain time and location requirements and can't be considered for accreditation. If this is the case, the ADA requires that the camp still meet the guidelines set forth by the American Camping Association.

If you're researching a camp and notice that it is not ACA accredited, ask why. If it's because they the camp does meet the standards for location and length of program, ask if it still works to maintain ACA guidelines. Almost any diabetes camp will be properly accredited. Beware of any camp that is not.

Safety record

All camps are subject to mishaps and accidents. It's the nature of the operation. A broken leg, a scraped knee—

these are the types of problems that commonly happen at any camp. Continuous problems related to improper diabetes management, such as frequent bouts with hypoglycemia and rampant blood sugars, are not typical of a well-run camp. Any camp with a history of these problems should be avoided.

Talk with the director about the camp's past safety record. You'll find that most camps have a surprisingly clean history, with very few diabetes-related problems. The camp director should be open and willing to talk about the camp's safety record and not afraid to mention any accidents that may have arisen over the years. In an outdoor environment with lots of kids running and playing all day long, something's bound to happen. Be wary of directors and counselors who try to skirt the issue, or say outright that they've never had a problem, because it's probably not true. Every camp has suffered a mishap over the years, unless it just recently opened.

4

The Application Process

After you've chosen a camp, it's time to start the application process. You should get the ball rolling as early as possible; if you can, begin in January or February for the upcoming summer. Some camps offer diabetes camps for only one or two weeks of the summer, so by the time May rolls around, it may well be too late.

Following is a step-by-step rundown of the application process you'll probably encounter. Each camp has its own procedures, but the overall process will be similar to the one described here. If you ever have any questions about the application process, contact your American Diabetes Association

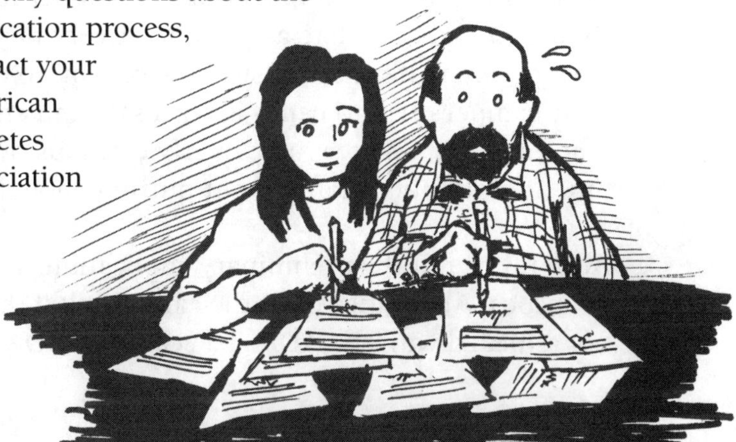

representative or the camp itself. Guesswork can sometimes lead to misleading or false information, which can spell trouble down the line. Always err on the side of caution.

Contact the ADA

If you've decided which camp you're interested in, you've probably already contacted either the local ADA office or the camp itself. If not, now's the time to do so. Within a couple of weeks, you should receive a preliminary application and some information about the camp. Sometimes a camp will just send promotional material until you express interest in the camp, other times they'll send an application only.

The first application you receive will not be the one that determines your camper's status at camp. This is merely to get basic information about you and your camper and to show that you are indeed interested in the camp. For the most part, it will just ask for simple contact information, such as name, age, how long your child has had diabetes, who to contact in case of an emergency, and whether or not you're interested in financial assistance.

When filling out the application, remember to be as thorough and complete as possible. Every piece of information, no matter how basic, is necessary to ensure that your camper's trip to camp is both safe and enjoyable. Once again, it's better to be overly cautious by putting too much information than by not putting enough.

After filling out the preliminary application, send it back to your local ADA office or to the camp itself if the camp is not affiliated with the ADA. The camp or ADA will process your application and make sure it is complete. They may contact you if additional information is needed, but this is unusual with first applications. You'll then move on to step two in the application process—filling out the packet.

The Packet

Soon after you send the first application, you'll receive a thick packet in the mail containing a variety of forms, from medical forms to the types of food your camper prefers. You'll also receive a variety of informational packets and documents. It will probably all seem a little overwhelming at first, but camps need to be as thorough as possible to ensure the safety of the campers. Below you'll find descriptions of the kinds of things you'll find in the packet. *(For examples of these forms, see Appendix B in the back of the book.)*

- **Medical form.** This one is probably the most daunting; luckily, your child's physician has to fill it out, not you. Unfortunately, the doctor's office sometimes neglects to complete the form and send it to the camp. So never assume that just because you gave the form to your physician that it was completed and sent in. You should call and check on its status, and it may even require a few gentle reminders. This is the most important document in the packet, and if the camp doesn't receive it in time, your camper may not make it to camp this summer.
- **Dietary form.** You'll have to fill out this one on your own. Any relevant information pertaining to your child's diet is noted here, from carbohydrate counts to foods that cause allergic reactions to the

types of food preferred. A regulated diet plan is an essential part of diabetes camp, and if the camp fixes food that your child won't or can't eat, it could wreak havoc on her blood sugars.

- **Information form.** This is an in-depth version of the preliminary application that you already filled out. In addition to things like emergency contact information, you'll be asked to give relevant information about behavioral issues or additional health concerns. Be sure to list anything the camp needs to know in order to care for your child properly.
- **Scholarship form (optional).** If you mentioned that you were interested in financial assistance on your

Helpful Tips for Filling Out Applications

- Get the forms in early. It doesn't matter when you start looking if the forms are sent late.
- Write clearly, in dark ink. Forms are often photocopied and the dark ink makes the copies easier to read.
- Check that you have filled out the form completely. For instance, be sure to put area codes for all phone numbers. Camps receive applications from all across the country, so local information needs to be included.
- Include all pertinent information on the forms. If your child has been to this camp before, don't assume that counselors and staff members remember the information. Even if the counselors work with your child outside of camp, there may still be things they don't know or perhaps have forgotten.
- Don't assume your physician's office has sent in the medical form on time—check to make sure it was sent, and that the camp received it.

preliminary application, you'll probably receive a scholarship form with your packet (*see Appendix C for a sample scholarship form*). This form varies from camp to camp, but it will probably just ask for basic financial information, such as family income, expenditures, and any other financial assistance that you're receiving.

Don't leave anything out

It is absolutely necessary that you mention any health issues or behavioral problems your child has. Parents are sometimes afraid that if they include this information on the application, their child will run a greater risk of being disqualified from camp. This is not the case. In fact, omitting it can leave the staff unprepared, which could cause your child to be sent home. A good camp will use the information to make reasonable provisions for your child's visit. But they can't do this if they don't know what your child needs.

Sometimes it's information that you didn't even think of that creates problems. One family's recent experience highlights this. It was their son's first time at camp, and the parents contacted the local ADA office to apply. He was accepted, packed his bags, and headed to camp. But when they dropped him off, they found out there was a problem. It turns out that the camp did not use the type of meter the family used at home, but this was the only kind their son used. In fact, there were no meters of this kind on the campgrounds. Of course, all campers' blood sugars have to be tested. Luckily, they compromised and worked out an alternate plan using another meter, but the whole thing could have been avoided if the parents had just mentioned on his application that he only used one type of meter and lancing device.

Similarly, any religious observances/restrictions should also be noted. If he needs to attend Saturday evening

Mass, arrangements may need to be made. If he eats only kosher foods, the kitchen staff needs to know in advance. If there are issues concerning dancing, dress codes, or other customs, you should inform the staff beforehand.

Basically, any information that might require the camp to adjust its schedule or processes should be included in your application. If you're not sure about an issue, talk to your ADA representative or the camp director. They'll tell you what's standard and what is not.

Information packets

Along with the forms, you'll also receive information packets. Be sure to read over all of the information thoroughly. If you're not clear on anything, call the ADA office and ask about it. Following are some of the documents you may receive:

- a list of what to bring to camp (see chapter 5)
- camp rules and regulations
- camp procedures
- an invoice
- directions to the camp

After you've carefully read all of the information and filled out the forms (and made sure your doctor's office sent its form), send them back to the ADA or camp office and wait for them to contact you.

If there are additional health concerns, behavioral issues, or religious accommodations that need to be made, an ADA representative or a camp staff member will contact you to get further information. They will discuss which accommodations can be made and which cannot. Usually, you'll be surprised at how flexible the camps are.

If a Camper Isn't Accepted

Camps do not look for ways to disqualify potential campers; on the contrary, they want as many campers as possible to attend and have a good time. If campers have health concerns, behavioral issues, or religious accommodations that need to be made, the camp personnel will work with parents to determine if reasonable provisions can be arranged. Sometimes camps can modify program offerings for certain campers based on their unique needs and limitations, or may need to work with camper families to reach agreement about behavior, expectations, and consequences.

It is very important that you fully prepare the camp staff with all the necessary information about your child's health, emotional, and behavior issues, including sexual history and orientation, drug and alcohol use, and psychological concerns. Withholding complete information inhibits the camp's ability to adequately prepare for your child and may result in early dismissal of the child from camp if the health or safety of your camper, other campers, or camp personnel is in danger. When parents identify health, behavior, and psychological concerns a camp representative will contact you to discuss how reasonable provision may be made for your camper. Parents and camp personnel together will determine if and how your child can be reasonably accommodated in the camp setting with the primary interest being the health and safety of all campers and camp personnel.

Keep in mind that the main reason most campers are not accepted to camp has nothing to do with behavior issues or health concerns; it has to do with capacity. Camps can only accept so many campers, so the earlier you get started the better.

You're Ready to Go

Once the camp has processed your application and made sure that all of the information is correct and complete, you'll probably get a notice that your child has been accepted to camp. Now it's time to gear up and get ready.

5

Packing Your Bags

Sometime during the application process, the camp director or a local ADA representative will mail you a list of the things you need to bring to camp. These lists vary from camp to camp, depending on the type of camp and the focus of the activities. For instance, you wouldn't need as much for a day camp as you would for a resident camp, since you're not staying the night and you'll probably be much closer to home.

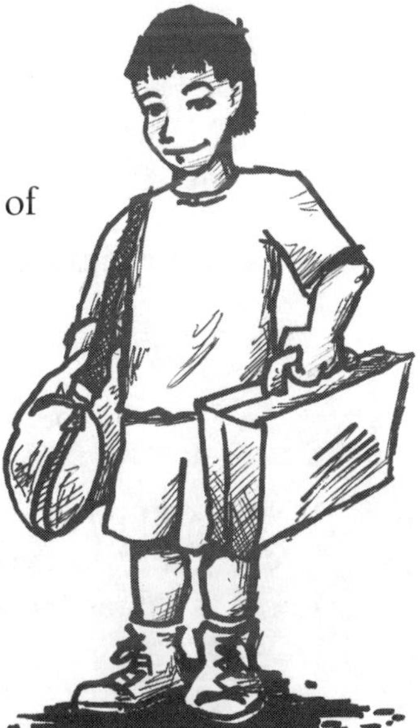

What to Bring

If the camp doesn't provide a list of things to bring, talk to the camp director about what items you need. Most resident-camp lists will look something like this:

- Sleeping bag or bedroll/pillow

- Towels, washcloth
- Shorts, jeans, slacks (if there's horseback riding, long pants are usually required)
- Shirts
- Socks
- Hat
- Tennis shoes, walking shoes
- Underwear
- Swimsuit
- Rain gear
- Jacket, sweater, or sweatshirt
- Pajamas
- Flashlight and extra batteries
- Bag for dirty clothes
- Camera/film (optional)
- Medication **not** related to diabetes (all drugs will need to be kept with the medical staff)
- Toiletries—soap, shampoo, etc. (nonaerosol)
- Sunscreen (nonaerosol)
- Insect repellent (nonaerosol)

If your camp has a particular focus, such as sports or overnight hikes, you'll probably need to bring additional items (such as backpacks or sports equipment).

Diabetes-related medical supplies
Medical supplies related to diabetes care are not on the list above because many diabetes camps supply them for you. But whether they do or not, it's always best to consult your physician to see what you will need, and then check whether these items are provided. Remember, if your camper requires anything that is not standard at the camp, be sure to let the camp director and your ADA representative know well ahead of time.

What Not to Bring

Camps discourage kids from bringing any item that may hinder them from fully participating in the camp experience. Remember, part of the reason your child is attending camp is to interact with others and to feel less isolated in their diabetes. Sometimes our electronic toys are a kind of crutch that we turn to whenever we're bored—instead of inventing some new game or just talking with others, we go into our own little computerized world. So anything that gets in the way of the process of making friends, even a book, may be frowned upon. Check with your camp to see what their policy is.

"A lot of counselors don't like their campers bringing radios, but I don't really have a problem with it, as long as they don't bring headphones. If they play it quietly, it gives them something to do at night before they go to sleep. Of course, if everybody brings a radio and everybody wants to listen to something different, then there can be a problem. It can also be a learning experience. Coming to an agreement on what to listen to and when to listen to it helps them learn to work together."

Counselor, Kansas City ADA Diabetes Camp at Camp Shawnee

For Kids Only:
Pack Your Bags, You're Going to Camp!

So you've been accepted and you're ready to go to camp. You can't wait to begin this cool adventure. But first it's time to pack your bags.

The problem is, you've never been to camp before, so what do you need to bring? The answer is: Not as much as you think! In fact, most campers bring way too much stuff. You're just going to be gone for a week or two. If you can't fit everything into two good-sized bags, you've probably overpacked.

Also keep in mind that one of the great things that camp offers is a chance to connect with nature. So leave the electronics at home. If you spend most of your time at camp glued to a Gameboy, you might just as well have saved the money and stayed home on the couch.

Leave behind anything that will keep you from being a part of the camp experience. Diabetes camp is a way for kids to connect with their environment and to connect with one another. If you bring things that keep you from taking advantage of this, you've missed the best part of camp.

What kinds of things are we talking about? It depends. Some camps even frown on books. It sounds a little crazy, but it is true that when you're reading a book, you're not taking part in the things going on around you. You can't talk to others, take part in activities, or experience all the fun that the camp has to offer. You're at camp to do new things. Take advantage of it!

Just about anything electronic should probably stay at home. Most counselors don't mind if you bring a portable radio to listen to at night while you're in your bunk, but that's usually about as far as it goes.

Some things you should probably leave at home include:

- Video games
- Cell phones (don't worry, if there's an emergency, you'll be able to reach your parents)
- Portable DVD players
- Portable TVs
- Laptop computers
- Puzzles and one-player games

Try to keep toys to a minimum. A few action figures, small stuffed animals, or some Hotwheels would be fine, but not a backpack full of them. Cards and compact, multiplayer games are usually okay. They give your bunk-house mates something to do together before you go to bed.

Basically, try not to bring anything that's going to exclude you from the rest of the camp. A no-book policy may be a little extreme, but the idea behind it makes sense. Talk to the other campers, talk to your counselors, take a walk in the woods with some friends, and participate in all of the activities. Make the most out of camp, and it will be an experience you'll never forget!

6

For Parents and Kids

What to Expect at Camp

By now, you've chosen a camp and have a pretty good idea about what it offers. You've talked with the staff, visited the site, and completed the application process. But your child may be wondering what is actually supposed to happen at camp—and what's *not* supposed to happen. And since your camper will be on her own once camp starts, we thought the following information should be addressed to both of you.

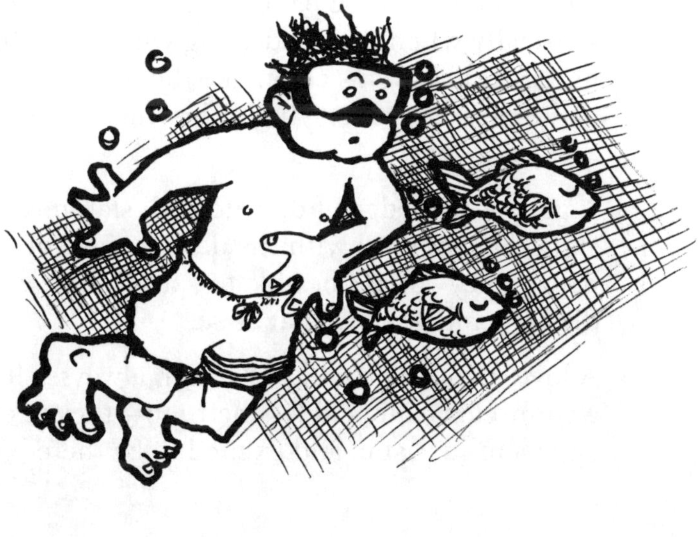

The Staff

A good staff can make a field trip to an abandoned parking lot seem like an adventure. They're the backbone of the camp. So how do you know you're in the hands of qualified professionals and not a bunch of uninterested part-timers?

What to expect

- Experience. Most good counselors get rehired year after year. The best counselors have a gift for working with kids, and camp directors snap them up quickly. If this is a counselor's first year, he should at least have been to camp as a kid. If they've had no experience whatsoever with camp or working with kids, this will probably be a learning experience.
- An ability to communicate well with kids and teenagers. A counselor may be the most caring person in the world, but it's wasted if they can't communicate well.
- A patient, positive, and caring disposition. Staff members need to be patient and understanding, especially when they're dealing with issues like homesickness. This can make the difference between a camper staying or leaving. Or returning again next year.
- A good knowledge of diabetes. All staff members should be familiar with the danger signs of diabetes. They should be able to spot trouble and handle any emergencies that arise.
- A love of kids and camp. You can always tell when a counselor really enjoys their job—they're energetic, enthusiastic, and excited to be there.

What to watch out for

- Inexperience with diabetes camp or diabetes. If you're at camp and you observe that your counselor or the supervising staff doesn't know much about diabetes, talk to the camp director or ADA representative about it.
- An impatient and short-tempered attitude. Being in charge of kids day in and day out can take a toll on just about anyone, and there are bound to be times when a counselor loses his cool. But these should be isolated instances. Counselors should never be quick to yell or reprimand a camper. Kids are going to make mistakes or do things they shouldn't, and a good counselor knows how to handle the situation calmly.
- Unnecessary disciplining. If campers do something they're not supposed to do, they are going to be disciplined—it's just a necessary part of camp. However, if it seems like there's more time spent disciplining than having fun, you might have a problem. Some counselors are stricter than others, but if you are constantly getting in trouble for little infractions, you should talk to the counselor or his supervisor *(see below)*.
- A lack of discipline. If campers are breaking the rules and out of control, it can ruin everyone's fun. Camp should not be a free-for-all.

> "I've only had a couple of counselors I didn't like. One was too crabby and she wouldn't wake up at night if we had a problem. The other one was too quiet; she wouldn't tell us what to do."
>
> **Camper, Age 10**

What to do if there's a problem

It can be hard to report a problem with the staff. You might be afraid that you'll get into trouble for talking to someone about it, or that the situation will just get worse. But no matter how scary it may be, you need to talk to the camp director about the problem. A well-run camp will deal with the situation in private and go to great lengths to see that the problem is resolved. Being a counselor is a job just like any other, and if a counselor continues to do things that aren't acceptable, they can lose their job. If you feel there is a problem, talk with the camp director. They will tell you what you need to do and will make sure that someone addresses the situation.

Other Campers

Being around other campers with diabetes is one of the greatest things about going to diabetes camp. You have the chance to establish close friendships, but you probably won't get along with every camper. And sometimes, other campers can be a big problem. You should expect the following from them:

- Honesty
- Respect for the property of others
- A willingness to participate in group activities
- The desire to have a good time
- Courtesy (it may not come naturally, but there should at least be an effort)

If you aren't getting along with another camper, try talking to them to see what the problem is. Most disputes are based on misunderstandings. Maybe they misunderstood something you did or said, or maybe you misunderstood them. If this doesn't seem to help, avoid the person as much as possible and try to still have fun with the other friends you've made. If the problem continues to interfere with your own good time, report the behavior to your counselor. Don't worry; you're not being a snitch. You're merely reporting what you feel is bad behavior.

A good counselor will sit down with both campers in question and talk with them, see where the problem is stemming from, and try to figure out a solution. The main thing is to not let trouble with another camper keep you from having a good time at camp. And believe it or not, a lot of campers who didn't get along at first eventually turn out to be best friends.

You won't win any friends if you report every minor incident, but if another camper's behavior is dangerous or destructive, you need to speak to a counselor about it. If the counselor is unable to resolve the problem, you may need to speak with the camp director or your parents. It is unlikely that you will encounter the following behavior, but if you do, it's good to know in advance that you do not have to put up with it. Serious issues that you may need to speak to a counselor about include:

- Dangerous or destructive behavior
- Theft
- Dishonesty
- Ridicule
- Threats or actual abuse, whether physical or verbal
- Constant attempts to make other people's camp experience unpleasant
- Not sticking to diabetes management guidelines

Activities

Activity schedules at camps vary widely. Some camps have a busy schedule for each camper to follow, while others offer a variety of activities from which to choose. We can't really discuss exactly which activities to expect from camp, since each one is different. Besides, at this point, you should already have a pretty good idea of the activities that your camp offers. However, we can give you some things to look for in how these activities are run and the nature of the activities offered. Camp activities should:

- foster a sense of accomplishment and teamwork.
- bring campers together in a fun and enriching environment.
- be well supervised.

Camp activities should not:

- put the campers at risk of injury or exhaustion.
- exclude certain campers unless the activity is voluntary (and special provisions have been made for excluded campers).

Facilities

Standards for the facilities vary, depending on the camp. For example, a day camp at a local church is probably going to be pretty safe and is close enough to medical help that it wouldn't pose much of a danger to campers. But a camp located deep in the woods, away from hospitals and emergency facilities, will need to have more ser-

Blood-Sugar Levels at Camp

Kids at camp will probably be much more active than they are at home, and this will dramatically affect their blood sugar levels. As a result, tight control at camp might be hard to achieve and could even be dangerous. With a long day of running, swimming, and climbing ahead of them, high blood sugars in the morning might help prevent lows throughout the day. Blood sugars will more than likely move in and out of target ranges, but in the long run, a healthy balance will be maintained (just take a look at their A1c levels). By learning how to keep blood sugars in a healthy range, children will be better prepared outside of camp for unexpected changes and periods of high activity, so this strategy can also educate campers.

vices and supplies on hand to ensure campers' safety. Although you visited the facilities and made your own inspections before choosing a camp, things may have changed since you last visited. Campers can expect the buildings and living quarters to be:

- cleaned on a regular basis.
- safe and free from dangerous materials that could cause burns, cuts, or other injuries.
- structurally sound.
- able to support emergency situations.
- capable of withstanding the elements, such as wind and rain.
- able to keep out wild animals.

Keep in mind that there is a wilderness factor involved if the camp is located in a natural setting. Facilities should

> "I didn't want to come to camp because I thought it was going to be just like a hospital, only dirty. I'm so glad I came, though. I've been coming for years and I have a great time every year. When I get too old to come as a camper, I want to be a counselor. I want to be a part of camp for as long as I can."
>
> **Camper, Age 14, Camp Nejeda**

be safe, but there are going to be things that you wouldn't find at home, especially if you live in an urban area. There will be spiders, poison ivy, bugs, and various woodland creatures, such as raccoons and mice. The facilities at a good camp will not pose a threat to the safety of the campers, but be prepared that the place will be a little rustic.

Use Common Sense

Many of these issues are ones that any camper or parent might expect and would be on the lookout for during their initial visit. If something would make a camper uncomfortable or keep him from having a good time, reject the camp. The best camps go to great lengths to make sure all of their campers have fun, and your own intuition will usually alert you if something is amiss. However, one thing that a lot of campers and parents don't anticipate has nothing to do with the other campers, the staff, or the facilities: homesickness.

7

Homesickness

It's bound to happen. If this is a camper's first trip to resident camp, she will probably feel homesick at some point. The intensity of it varies—some kids miss home terribly for a few minutes and then forget all about it; others think about home the entire time they're away. And it's almost impossible to predict how homesick a camper will be. Sometimes, the friendly, extroverted camper that you think would be the last person to get homesick can't stop thinking about home, while the shy, quiet kid ends up having fun right from the start.

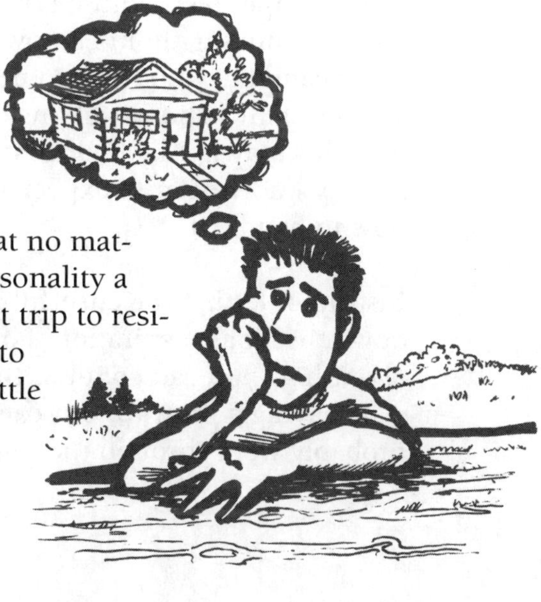

But it's a safe bet that no matter what type of personality a camper has, her first trip to resident camp is going to result in at least a little homesickness. The thing to remember is that the homesickness will pass and that there are ways to cope with what seems like an unbearable longing for home.

A lot of campers get embarrassed when they get homesick, which just compounds the feelings of loneliness and isolation. They look around and see the other campers enjoying themselves, but all they can think about is the end of the week, when mom and dad will show up to bring them home. Naturally, this makes them feel like they're the only one experiencing this, which makes them feel even more alone, and the whole thing spirals into a vicious cycle. And no matter how much you try to prepare them, in the end it's the children who have to deal with it, on their own. So the rest of this chapter is addressed to them.

For Kids Only: Who, Me? Homesick?

When your parents are bugging you to clean your room and your brothers and sisters are getting on your nerves, it's hard to believe you would ever feel homesick. But every camper feels a little homesick at some point. So if you start missing home, know that you're not alone. Even those campers who seem to be having the most fun probably feel a little homesick inside, despite how they look. And this may not be their first trip to camp, so they may already know what to expect and have a better idea of how to handle it.

Instead of letting the cheerful attitude of others get you down, use it as inspiration. Look at them to get ideas about how you can conquer the homesick feeling and start having a great time at camp. Remember, they probably went through the same things you're going through now and learned to handle it in lots of different ways.

Talk about it

One of the best ways to cope with your longing for home is to talk to someone about it. Your first instinct may be to bottle it up and not let anyone know how you feel. But if you talk about it with other campers, you'll be surprised at how many of them are feeling it too or have felt it before. They can tell you how they handled the situation and give you pointers on how you can make it better. Sometimes it's enough just knowing that they felt it too, because you automatically feel less alone. Plus, seeing that they have overcome the feeling and are having a great time shows that you can do it too!

It's understandable if you don't feel like talking with the other campers about what you're feeling. So talk to a counselor or staff member instead. A good counselor can help you get over your homesickness and put you on the road to enjoying yourself. Most counselors were campers once too, so it's a pretty safe bet that they know exactly

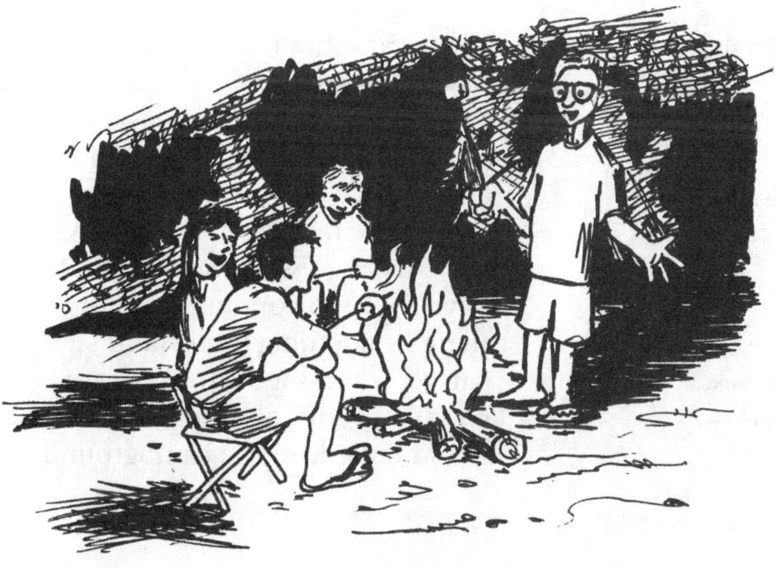

what you're going through. Another option is to find someone else who seems to be lonely and to make friends with him. They may be feeling the same things you are, so it could help both of you.

Don't Call Your Parents!

> "Almost every year there's a camper who gets really homesick; it's normal. But every time we help them get through it, and almost nobody ever goes home. Just recently we had a camper that was really down, but I talked him through it and he was so proud that he didn't cry or ask to go home or call his parents. He just stuck with it and ended up having a really good time."
>
> **Tony, Counselor, Camp Nejeda**

Believe it or not, the worst thing you can do if you're homesick is to call home. If you call within the first couple of days of camp, you're almost guaranteed to ask to go home early. Any counselor, camp director, or staff member will tell you that once a camper calls home, it's all over. So keep in mind that when you're feeling like you just can't take it anymore, but your counselor doesn't want you to call home, she's not just being mean. She's doing you a favor. She wants to help you work through your homesickness so you'll stay at camp and see how much fun it is.

This is another reason why cell phones aren't a good idea at camp. A cell phone makes it too easy to call home and have mom and pop come and get you. If you feel you need a cell phone in case of emergency, don't worry; the staff will always have a way to communicate. If there's something important, staff can relay messages. You'll never be completely out of touch with the world outside of the campground.

This may sound a little strict for a week or two of fun in the sun. But it's just a precaution that camps take to make sure you end up having a good time. It may sound harsh, but it works, and you'll thank your counselors for it later.

For Parents Only:
The Same Goes for You

The first time the kids are away from home can be pretty tough on parents, too. The urge to call your kid to check on him or just to hear his voice can be pretty strong. However, it's an urge that you should resist. Calling your child at camp can actually make things worse, especially if he's feeling just a little bit homesick. Calling staff to check up on your camper, on the other hand, is perfectly fine.

If your camper does call you from camp, resist the urge to let him come home right away. It's easy to give in to a child who seems distraught and frightened, but try to reassure him that he can still have fun at camp and if he comes home early, he'll be really disappointed later on. Remind him that if he can just hang in there for a few days, he'll end up having a great time!

Camp can be one of the most enriching experiences of a young person's life, and you want to encourage this step toward independence. Write supportive letters that will arrive during the week your child's at camp. Make opening day separation positive and relatively short; don't linger around and keep your child from meeting other campers. In fact, it's best to introduce your child to other campers and staff right away. At home, be strong and resist the urge to pick up the phone. And if it helps, just remember, you paid for this camp!

But if he's still homesick a few days later and his counselor thinks he's really having a hard time, you might want to let him come home. Some kids do get severely homesick, and it doesn't get any better as the week goes on. (*See below, "If It Doesn't Work Out, There's Always Next Year" for advice on leaving camp early.*)

Ways to Cope

So you can't call your parents, and they can't call you. You're staying at a new place miles from home. How do you cope with the homesickness you're feeling? Here are a few suggestions:

- ▲ Making friends is the easiest way to start having fun, so try interacting with the other campers more.
- ▲ Getting involved in all the new activities will help you focus on something else besides home.
- ▲ Staying busy keeps your mind off things—the more "down" time you have, the more you're going to think about home.

Homesickness can be worse at night, when you're in your bunk trying to fall asleep. To help with these times, try one of these suggestions:

- ▲ Write a letter home. Calling home isn't always the best idea, but there's nothing wrong with writing a letter to let everyone know you're thinking about them. Plus, the thought of getting a letter back can give you something to look forward to during the week.

- Try writing in a journal or a diary or drawing a picture. It doesn't matter if you're not the best writer or artist in the world. Just getting it out of your system can be a big help.
- Make the most of your day so that when bedtime comes, you're ready to fall asleep. If you're not sleepy when the lights go out, lying there can be torture. On the other hand, if you're worn out from a long day of activity, you'll fall asleep before you have time to feel lonely!

These are just a few suggestions. You know best what will make you feel better. Talking to counselors can also give you some good ideas. Their job is to help you and make sure you have fun, and they know how to do it better than anyone else does. Trust them and let them help you, and you'll find that in no time you'll be having a blast!

If It Doesn't Work Out, There's Always Next Year

Every so often, it doesn't work out for a camper and the best option really is to go home early. If a camper truly feels that he or she can't handle being away from home, the camp director won't stand in your way. Sometimes, it's because you weren't really ready for camp in the first place. Other times, a difficult situation at home makes it hard to be away from the family just then. Or perhaps the camp is just too different from what you thought it would be.

If this happens to you, don't worry about it. You haven't failed at anything, and no harm has been done. Sometimes things just don't work out. The main thing is to not let this one bad experience spoil the way you look at camps forever. Many campers who weren't ready the first summer have such a great time the next time around that they come back year after year. In fact, now that you know what to expect, you'll be a lot better prepared for your next week away from home.

Camp can be a great experience for campers, counselors, and everyone involved. Don't let this one bad experience keep you from many summers of fun!

8

Traditional Camps

For some families, a traditional summer camp, one not specifically focused on diabetes, is the best option. Maybe there aren't any diabetes camps in your area, maybe your child wants to try something that a diabetes camp doesn't offer, or maybe your camper wants to be with friends who are going to a traditional, nondiabetes summer camp.

Many parents feel nervous sending their child to a traditional camp. They fear that the camp will not be able to handle the added responsibility of diabetes. But while this choice does entail more responsibility on your part, and on the part of the camp you have chosen, it can be a fun, safe alternative to diabetes camps.

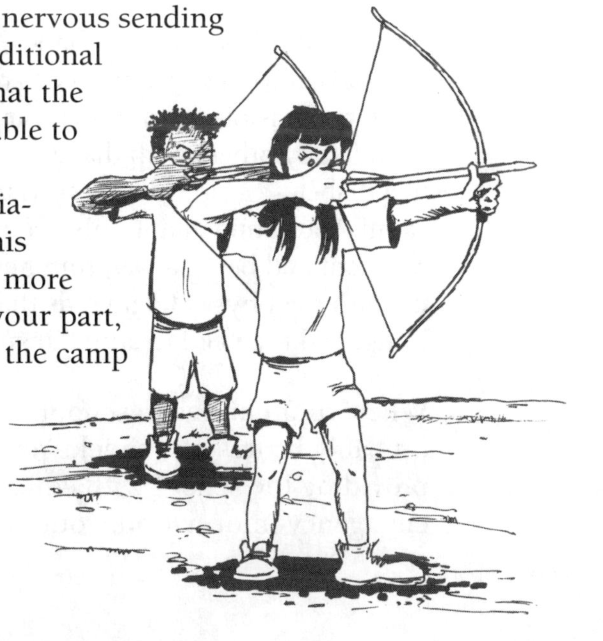

Traditional camps today are more inclusive than ever, and they are usually happy to accept children with special needs. However, you will need to ensure that the camp is prepared to adequately care for your child. Camps will go a long way to accommodate you, but personnel have not been specifically educated in diabetes care. They probably will not have the supplies and medicine a child with diabetes needs, so it's up to you to provide them. But before we get into what you need to bring, what to let the camp know, and so forth, you need to decide whether your camper is ready for a traditional camp.

Is Your Child Ready for a Traditional Camp?

Sending a child with diabetes to a traditional camp brings unique concerns. Will the child be able to handle his own diabetes care so far away from home? Will she be able to tell counselors when she's having a problem? Will he be able to adjust to the environment safely? These are some of the important questions you need to ask yourself.

If your child has attended diabetes camp, the switch to a traditional camp might take some adjustment. She will be more responsible for her own care and will not be surrounded by others with diabetes. On the other hand, going to a diabetes camp is the best way to prepare for a traditional camp. Your child is not only accustomed to the camp environment and being away from her parents, she is also familiar with the physical demands that full days of activities bring, and the need to adjust insulin dosages accordingly.

When your child is in school, a nondiabetes camp will probably be less of a shock. You're already familiar with providing the school with educational materials and emergency information. Your child has learned to take some responsibility for her own care when away from home. And although camp is not the same as school (kids are farther away and are more active), your child has already been around adults who may know less about diabetes than she does.

If your child has not yet started school, still needs you to visit her often during the school day to care for her, or is reluctant to take responsibility for her own care, a traditional camp is probably not the best place to start. Children with diabetes should attend diabetes camp at least once before they move on to traditional camps. Deciding whether or not your child is ready for a traditional camp can be a tough call. If you feel she is ready and your child feels that she is ready, it's time to start making preparations.

Before Heading to Camp

Visit the doctor

The first thing a child must do is to visit his doctor. Your child's activity level at camp will be much higher than it is at home or at school, so insulin doses will have to be adjusted to compensate. Your doctor will be able to suggest changes to the insulin dose and how much your child will need to alter his or her diabetes-care routine.

You should also ask your diabetes care team to contact the nurse at camp to go over your child's diabetes care. You will also need to do some educating of the camp staff yourself, but your doctor will be best prepared to give advice and explain the diabetes-care regimen. She can explain insulin administration, blood-glucose monitoring, and other aspects of care from a professional standpoint.

Pack your supplies

Unlike diabetes camp, a nondiabetes camp will not have diabetes supplies on hand. Your diabetes-care team can tell you what you'll need, but it will be your responsibility to make sure your child has everything while he is away from home.

Pack a diabetes backpack or cooler that your child can keep with him at all times while he's at camp. The contents will vary, but they should probably include the following:

- meter and extra meter strips
- extra snacks, such as cookies, granola bars, and crackers
- Fruit drinks or Gatorade
- Packets of frosting or sugar
- emergency contact information
- pump supplies (if your child is on a pump)

Make sure the backpack or cooler is portable and not too bulky. He might be reluctant to carry it around if he thinks it will make him stand out or be labeled as different, so it might help if he thinks it's cool-looking. Diabetes is nothing to be ashamed of, and if he just explains why he is carrying this stuff around, most of the other campers will be intrigued by it. And he may need to be reminded that not having his supplies or medication at the right time can pose a serious threat to his health.

What the Camp Needs

Basically, the camp needs anything that will help them better care for your child. You don't want to inundate them with so many requests and books and pamphlets that they start to resent your child and diabetes in general. But it's good to talk to the staff, the nurse, and the person in charge of meals and nutrition to let everybody know what they need to do to keep your child safe. Much of the information you provided when your child first started attending school would be suitable for camp.

Many parents like to send a short video that gives a brief description of diabetes and the warning signs of hypoglycemia and other possible disorders. Others like to send books and pamphlets on the subject. If possible, try to keep educational materials brief. Most people won't mind watching a 15-minute video, but a 300-page book usually just collects dust. Appendix D of this book has a list of the warning signs for hypoglycemia and hyperglycemia that you should copy and send to camp. The ADA also has a kit of materials about diabetes you can download from the website.

On the list of emergency numbers, you should include contact information for:

- You, your spouse, or other caregiver (work, home, and cell phone numbers)
- Your child's diabetes doctor or primary care provider
- Members of the diabetes-care team
- Other family members or friends

Nurses and nutrition

The camp nurse will be the one primarily responsible for your child's diabetes care at camp, so you should create a good rapport with her and include her in your preparations. In addition, your doctor or a member of your diabetes-care team should talk with her. The nurse will probably be familiar with diabetes and what the condition entails, but it's important to let her know specific details of your child's care. For example, if your child will only draw blood from a certain place, she needs to know. If your child is on a pump, the nurse may not be familiar with how it works. Go over with her what needs to be done and how to handle pump materials.

Your child also has different nutritional concerns than the other campers. Whoever is in charge of meals needs to know what your child needs for good nutrition and meal planning. Make sure they understand that it's important to provide food your child will eat, since not eating can pose a serious threat to your child's health. Having a registered dietician talk with the meal-planning department might be a good idea as well.

Try Not to Worry

Try not to worry if your child is attending a traditional summer camp. Camp in general is a great way for children with diabetes to develop a sense of independence, and moving on to a nondiabetes camp can be a big step in furthering this sense of confidence and self-reliance. Remember that your child is learning valuable things about themselves and their diabetes care.

Unlikely, But Possible

It's hard to imagine that a camp would deny a camper admission based on medical concerns, and luckily, incidents like this are few and far between. However, if your camper was not accepted to a nondiabetes camp, and you believe it was due to his or her medical condition, you're entitled to certain legal rights. If you feel you have been discriminated against because of diabetes, contact an ADA advocate by calling 1-888-DIABETES.

9

Evaluating the Camp

Was It Worth It?

A camper usually knows whether or not the camp was good. If he or she had fun (which is almost always the case), that's a pretty good sign that things went well. Sometimes, however, the experience was not a positive one, or was only a partial success. Here are some questions to help you evaluate it, determine what the problems were, and find things you might want to address down the line.

Did He Do His Part?

First, you need to determine how much your child gave to the experience. No camp can provide a good time if he won't let it. It's up to him to participate in the activities and opportunities that camp offers, so before you

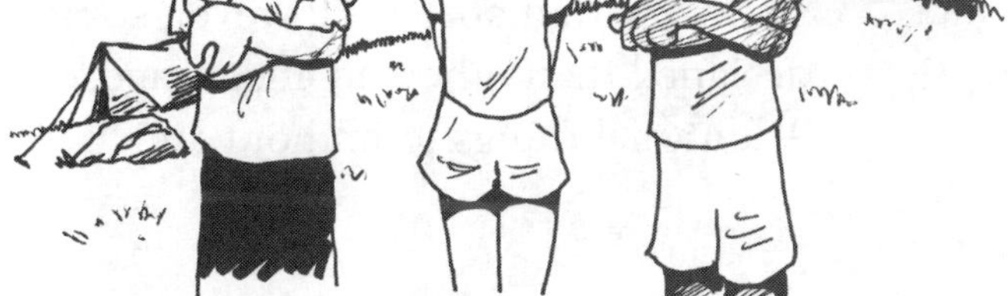

can evaluate the camp, you'll need to ask him the following questions:

- Did he participate in the activities that were offered?
- Did he try new things, maybe even activities that he hadn't planned on participating in?
- Did he talk with the other campers and try to meet new people?
- Did he listen to the staff when they had advice to give?
- Did he follow the rules of the camp?

If your son answered no to more than one of these questions, chances are he didn't really try to have a good time. Campers and the staff need to work together, and if a child doesn't fully participate, he's bound to be bored.

Evaluating the Camp

Of course, the camp has to keep its part of the bargain. Sometimes camps don't meet the children's (or parents') expectations. To see if your camp made the grade, find out the answer to these questions.

Did he get an opportunity to meet other kids with diabetes?

At diabetes camp, you're sure to meet other kids and staffers with diabetes. However, some camps are better designed than others to encourage kids to mingle. Additional things to find out are:

- Did he have free time to hang out with other campers?
- Did the camp organize activities so that he had to work with other campers to accomplish a goal?
- Was everything so structured or so unstructured that you barely got to know the other camper's names?

If a camp is too structured, campers don't get much time to be together on their own time. If it's not structured enough, kids don't get a chance to meet one another because it's too chaotic. A good camp should strike the proper balance between planned activities and freedom to give campers opportunities to make friends and have fun.

> "I've made so many friends at camp and I'll probably have them for the rest of my life. That's why I come to camp."
>
> **Camper, Age 12, ADA Camp at Camp Green Lane**

Did it help his self-esteem?

This is a tricky question. It's hard to gauge just what kind of impact a camp can have on a camper's confidence and self-esteem. But whether or not there were noticeable results, confidence building should be intricately woven into the fabric of the operation. Other things to find out are:

- Did the camp push you to achieve goals that you thought you couldn't accomplish?
- Did the camp help you to accomplish these goals?
- Did it recognize achievements with praise or some other reward?
- Were the counselors supportive and encouraging?
- Were you encouraged to try new things and learn new skills not related to your diabetes?

- Did the activities sometimes seem pointless or too competitive?
- Did the counselors put people down or have a negative attitude?
- Did you feel like a failure when you couldn't accomplish something?

Camps usually do an excellent job of building confidence and encouraging campers to achieve more than they expected of themselves. For campers, sometimes just being around others like themselves can be a big boost to their self-esteem and confidence.

Did he learn anything?

Your camper probably learned a lot at camp. If he didn't, it probably means that he didn't commit himself to learning something new. This doesn't mean that a camper should come back with a notebook full of facts they've learned over the course of the week. In fact, they may not be aware that they learned anything at all, because so much of the learning takes place outside of the traditional classroom. To find out more, you could ask:

- Were there scheduled educational activities?
- Did these activities encourage campers to participate?
- Were the counselors helpful and did they share their knowledge of diabetes?

> "Before I came to camp, my mom always had to change my pump site. Now I do."
>
> **Camper, Age 13**

Did he have fun?

This is one of the most important questions to ask, and the one that needs no explanation. If he had fun, he knows it. If he didn't have fun, he probably has a pretty good idea why. Encourage your child to explain why it wasn't fun and to pinpoint the problems that kept him from having fun.

The Biggest Indicator of Success

The biggest indicator that a camper had a good time and that her trip was a success is that she wants to go back next year. She probably met people that she wants to see again, and the activities helped her to feel more confident. There may be things that she didn't like, or certain issues that you feel you need to address, but if she wants to go back, it was worth all the time and money.

If she answered no to some of the questions above, she may not have had a very good time at camp. This could be because there was a camper that she didn't get along with or because one of the counselors was too strict. Maybe the activities weren't what she expected, or the camp focused too much on things she didn't care for. But even if she found that she didn't like camp at all, try not to give up on it completely. There are lots of different camps available with many different approaches. Just because she didn't like one camp doesn't mean she won't like another. Camps are designed to be fun and entertaining for all kinds of kids. There's bound to be a camp out there that's just right for your child.

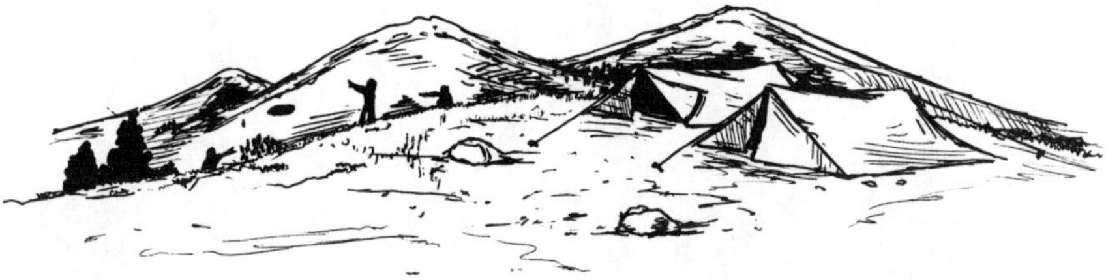

APPENDIX A

Diabetes Camp List

Following is a partial list of diabetes camps across the United States, including information about the type of camp and who to contact. Dates and pricing are not listed due to yearly changes and updates. For more information concerning camps in your area, pricing, and schedules, please visit *www.diabetes.org/wizdom/liveitup/camp. shtml.* There you'll find up-to-date information on a wide variety of camps across the country. And for more information and lists of additional camps, check the Diabetes Camping Association at *www. diabetescamps.org.*

NAME OF CAMP (listed alphabetically by state)	TYPE OF CAMP
ALABAMA	
Camp Seale Harris	Various
ALASKA	
Camp Kushtaka Located in Snug Harbor near Coppers Landing, this program combines the fun of outdoor activities with daily diabetes management education.	Resident Camp
ARIZONA	
Camp AZDA Located in Friendly Pines Camp in the tall plains of the Bradshaw Mountains, six miles outside Prescott. While campers learn more each day about diabetes management, the main goal of camp is fun. Daily activities include swimming, tennis, western riding, water boarding, wagon rides, archery, fishing, and hiking. A challenge course and rock climbing are available for older campers.	Resident Camp
ARKANSAS	
Camp Aldersgate *Little Rock*	Resident Camp
CALIFORNIA	
Camp Conrad-Chinnock	Resident Camp Operated by the Diabetic Youth Services, Inc.
Camp Wana Cura	Day Camp
COLORADO	
Camp Colorado Located at Eagle Lake Camp, just 45 minutes north-west of Colorado Springs and adjacent to Pikes Peak National Forest. Resident Camp, Wilderness Camp, Bike Camp, and Equestrian Camp are offered.	Resident Camp
CONNECTICUT Please refer to *Camp Carefree* in *New Hampshire*	

NAME OF CAMP (listed alphabetically by state) (*continued*)	TYPE OF CAMP
FLORIDA **Florida's Diabetes Camp**	Multi-week Day, Resident, and Weekend events for children, their siblings, friends, and families.
Jada Camp Jada features a variety of new and exciting activities that are sure to send campers home with smiles and many stories to tell. Thursday night is Parent's Night, with dinner provided for campers and their families.	Day Camp
GEORGIA Please refer to the *Florida* or *South Carolina* camps	
HAWAII **He Ola Ke Keiki** Started in 1968, the camp provides youth with a wholesome camping experience as well as the opportunity to learn diabetes management skills.	Resident Camp
IDAHO Please refer to camps in *Montana* or *Washington*	
ILLINOIS **Camp Can-Do** *Ridge Park, Chicago* The goal of this day camp program is to provide children with the opportunity to participate in recreational activities while developing independence and confidence in caring for their diabetes. Siblings and friends are welcome.	Day Camp
Camp Confidence *United Methodist Camp Grounds, Des Plaines* This camp strives to provide children with the opportunity to participate in entertaining activities while fostering independence and confidence in caring for their diabetes. Siblings and friends are welcome.	Day Camp

(*continued*)

NAME OF CAMP (listed alphabetically by state) (*continued*)	TYPE OF CAMP
ILLINOIS (*continued*)	
Camp Crossroads at Camp Tu-Endie-Wei *Elgin* This camp works to nurture independence and confidence in a safe, fun environment. Siblings and friends are welcome.	Day Camp
Camp Discovery *Butterfield Park District* Day camp program dedicated to providing children with the opportunity to participate in recreational activities while developing independence and confidence in caring for their diabetes. Siblings and friends are welcome.	Day Camp
Camp Granada This camp provides an opportunity for children with diabetes ages 8-16 to learn more about themselves and their diabetes in a fun-filled and safe camping environment. The program encourages self-management while providing appropriate medical supervision and allowing the best possible camper experience.	Resident Camp
Camp Kids	Day Camp
Teen Adventure Camp Camp is held at Covenant Point, located on the scenic shores of Hagerman Lake in Iron River, Michigan. Bus transportation is provided from two Chicagoland locations.	Resident Camp
Camp Triangle D Camp is held at YMCA Camp Duncan on Route 12 just north of Route 120 in Ingleside, Illinois.	Resident Camp
INDIANA	
Camp John Warvel With an emphasis on fun, Camp John Warvel offers a unique learning atmosphere for children with diabetes to acquire (according to their developmental levels) new skills in caring for their diabetes. Positive attitudes about diabetes and self-confidence in diabetes management are instilled through education, encouragement, and example.	Resident Camp

NAME OF CAMP (listed alphabetically by state) (*continued*)	TYPE OF CAMP
IOWA	
Camp Hertko Hollow Camp is held at the Des Moines YMCA Camp north of Boone, Iowa.	Resident Camp
KANSAS	
Camp Discovery Camp Discovery is in its 28th year of operation. It offers young people with diabetes the opportunity to have a fun and exciting summer experience while learning more about their diabetes self-management.	Resident Camp
Camp Ka-Di-Da-Ca Kansas Diabetes Day Camp is a special day camp for children ages 5-8 with diabetes, their siblings, and/or friends. Campers have the opportunity to swim, play games, make arts and crafts, and learn more about diabetes.	Day Camp
KENTUCKY	
Camp Hendon Held at Boy Scout Camp Crooked Creek next to Bernheim Forest near Sherpherdsville. Activities offered at camp include swimming, canoeing, wind surfing, astronomy, archery, riflery, volleyball, softball, nature hikes, and team-building courses.	Resident Camp
LOUISIANA	
Louisiana Lions Camp *Leesville*	Resident Camp
MAINE	
Please refer to *Camp Carefree* in *New Hampshire*	
MARYLAND	
Camp Glyndon at Lions Camp Merrick Located at Lions Camp Merrick in Charles County, Maryland, Glyndon offers a wide range of activities, including swimming, a challenge course, and drama.	Resident Camp
MASSACHUSETTS	
Clara Barton Camp	Resident Camp Operated by Clara Barton Camp

(*continued*)

NAME OF CAMP (listed alphabetically by state) (*continued*)	TYPE OF CAMP
MASSACHUSETTS (*continued*)	
Joslin Diabetes Camp	Resident Camp Operated by Joslin Diabetes Center
MICHIGAN	
Camp Midicha Camp Midicha is located on the YMCA Camp Copneconic property in Fenton, just south of Flint. Camp Midicha is a place where lifelong friends are made and all the kids have diabetes, so no one feels different. Along with swimming, canoeing, kayaking, and sports, Camp Midicha offers horseback riding, high ropes course, and crafts.	Resident Camp
MINNESOTA	
Camp Day Point The perfect introduction to camp, Day point is nonstop fun in a comfortable environment. Amid all the fun, campers gain independence, grow in confidence, discover new skills, and learn respect for others and for the outdoors.	Day Camp
Camp Needlepoint Camp Needlepoint programs encourage independence and self-management with appropriate medical supervision to ensure the best possible experience for every camper. Younger campers have fun in stable, structured activities, while older campers welcome the challenge of canoeing or sailing adventures.	Resident Camp
MISSISSIPPI	
Twin Lakes Diabetes Camp *Jackson*	Resident Camp
MISSOURI	
Camp Day Break	Day Camp
Camp Earthworks I & II	Two one-week sessions of day camp at two different locations.
Camp EDI	Resident Camp

NAME OF CAMP (listed alphabetically by state) (*continued*)	TYPE OF CAMP
Camp Redbird	Day Camp
Kansas City Diabetes Camp At Camp Shawnee The primary goal of Kansas City Diabetes Camp is to teach children with diabetes how to enjoy a healthy, active lifestyle.	Resident Camp
MONTANA	
Montana's Youth Retreat	Resident Camp
NEBRASKA	
Camp Hot Shots *Platte River State Park* This camp is located approximately 20 miles from Omaha and 30 miles from Lincoln. Camp Hot Shots provides a fun, safe, and educational environment for kids with diabetes.	Day Camp
NEVADA Please refer to camps in *New Mexico* and *Arizona.*	
NEW HAMPSHIRE	
Camp Carefree The mission of Camp Carefree is to provide a fun-filled, educational camping experience for children with diabetes that will help them to develop and maintain active, healthy lifestyles.	Resident Camp
NEW JERSEY	
Camp Nejeda	Resident Camp
NEW MEXICO	
Camp Challenge Camp Challenge is held at Camp Stoney near Santa Fe. Camping activities include swimming, sports, hiking, and a challenge ropes course.	Resident Camp
NEW YORK	
Camp Independence	Day Camp
Camp Sunshine Held at Rotary Camp Sunshine south of Rochester, the ADA program includes swimming, nature trails, fishing, and other camp activities offered in a rural setting.	Resident Camp

(*continued*)

NAME OF CAMP (listed alphabetically by state) (*continued*)	TYPE OF CAMP
NEW YORK (*continued*)	
DSG Day Camp	Day Camp
Camp Rainbow	Day Camp
NORTH CAROLINA	
Camp Enscore	Day Camp
Cumberland Day Camp	Day Camp
Camp Carolina Trails	Resident Camp
NORTH DAKOTA	
Camp Sioux	Resident Camp
Camp Sioux was founded in 1952 for children with insulin- dependent diabetes. Every summer, two week-long sessions allow campers to discover the joys and adventures of the rugged outdoors under the careful supervision of a highly skilled diabetes team.	
OHIO	
Camp Korelitz	
The Camp Korelitz program is designed to meet the diverse needs and interests of its campers. During the week, campers will participate in group and individual activities, including team sports, swimming, campfires, outdoor education, arts and crafts, drama, and archery.	Resident Camp
Camp Tokumto	
Cincinnati	Day Camp
At Camp Tokumto we believe that educational and recreational camping improves the lives of young people with diabetes, providing a creative opportunity to enhance their physical, emotional, and social well being.	
OKLAHOMA	
Please refer to camps in *Arkansas*.	
OREGON	
Please refer to camps in *Washington*.	
PENNSYLVANIA	
Camp Crestfield	Resident Camp

NAME OF CAMP (listed alphabetically by state) (*continued*)	TYPE OF CAMP
American Diabetes Association Camp for Kids at Camp Green Lane Located in Montgomery County, Pennsylvania, the camp offers a wide variety of activities, including swimming, a challenge course, drama, nature lore, hiking, arts and crafts, and diabetes education.	Resident Camp
RHODE ISLAND Please refer to *Camp Carefree* in *New Hampshire*.	
SOUTH CAROLINA **Adam Fisher**	Resident Camp
Camp Independence	Day Camp
SOUTH DAKOTA **Camp Gilbert** Camp is held at NeSoDak Camp on Lake Enemy Swim near Waubay, South Dakota. A special leadership program for high-school campers is offered. This camp is operated by the South Dakota Children's Specialty Clinics at Sioux Valley Hospital and University Medical Center.	Resident Camp
TENNESSEE **Rising Sun**	Resident Camp
Sugar Falls	Day Camp
TEXAS **Camp Bluebonnet**	Day Camp
Camp Rainbow *Houston* Held at the YMCA Camp Pine Tree property in Spring, Texas, Camp Rainbow offers swimming, arts and crafts, games, and other recreational activities.	Day Camp
Camp New Horizons North *Dallas*	Day Camp
New Horizons South *Dallas*	Day Camp

(*continued*)

NAME OF CAMP (listed alphabetically by state) (*continued*)	TYPE OF CAMP
TEXAS ***(continued)***	
Camp Aurora *Fort Worth*	Day Camp
Camp Sandcastle *Corpus Christi*	Day Camp
VERMONT Please refer *to Camp Carefree* in *New Hampshire.*	
VIRGINIA Please refer to camps in *North Carolina* and *Maryland.*	
WASHINGTON	
Camp Dudley Camp Dudley, owned and operated by the Yakima Family YMCA, is located on picturesque Clear Lake, off Route 12 near Naches, Washington. This unique, 3-day session offers kids exciting and fun camp activities including swimming, boating, arts and crafts, games, campfires, and cookouts.	Resident Camp
Camp Sealth Camp Sealth is owned and operated by the Seattle King County Council of Camp Fire USA. Campers choose either a 4- or 6-day session or attend both. Located in spectacular Vashon Island southwest of Seattle, Camp Sealth offers a wide variety of camp and specialty programs, such as creative dramatics, archery, kayaking, canoeing, wind surfing, and sailing.	Resident Camp
Camp Orkila Camp Orkila's 12-day program offers the adventure of a lifetime on beautiful Orcas Island in the San Juans. Owned and operated by the YMCA of Greater Seattle, camp Orkila offers popular camp activities such as team sports, swimming, kayaking, canoeing, sailing, crafts, and nature study. Campers also participate in the Adventure ropes course and climbing wall, archery, riflery, hiking, as well as a cruiser ride to a neighboring island for a camp out. Horseback riding is also available.	Resident Camp

NAME OF CAMP (listed alphabetically by state) (*continued*)	TYPE OF CAMP
Camp Fun in the Sun Camp Fun in the Sun is located on Lake Couer d'Arlene in Worley, Idaho, approximately 45 minutes from Spokane, Washington.	Resident Camp
WEST VIRGINIA Please refer to camps in *Ohio, Kentucky,* and *Pennsylvania.*	
WISCONSIN **Camp Lakota**	Resident Camp
WYOMING Please refer to *Camp Colorado* in *Colorado.*	

American Camping Association

The American Camping Association is the world's leading authority on camps. For over 90 years, they've worked to ensure quality and safety in the camp environment. Their accreditation is the standard among campgrounds across the country and around the globe. If you need any information on traditional, nondiabetes camps or camping in general, the ACA is an excellent source.

American Camping Association
5000 State Road 67 North
Martinsville, IN 46151-7902
Phone: 765-342-8456
Fax: 765-342-2065
Web: *www.acacamps.org*

APPENDIX B

Sample Application Packet

Following is a sample packet, similar to the one you would probably receive in the application process. A sample scholarship application can be found in Appendix C.

FORM NAME	FORM LETTER
■ Camper Application Form	(Form A 1, 2, 3)
■ Camper Information Form	(Form B)
■ Consent Form	(Form C)
■ Camp Nutrition Form	(Form D)
■ Camp/Parent Agreement on Camp Rules	(Form E)
■ Health History Form	(Form F)

PROSPECTIVE CAMPER

Form A1

CAMPER APPLICATION FORM

To be filled out by Parent or Guardian

Check One:

ADA Member Fee _____ Non-Member Fee ____ Campership Fee $15 _____

Membership# ____________________

(*Fee should be enclosed with application*)

Date ______/______/______ T-Shirt Size, Adults: S____M____ L____XL ____

Camper's Name: ____

Camper's Address: ____

City: ______________________ State: ______ Zip: __________ County: ______________

Home Phone: ( ) ____________________ Home

In case of emergency notify: ________________________ Phone# ( ) ______________

Mother or Guardian's Name: ____

Occupation: ____

Work Phone: ( ) ____________________ Home Phone: ( ) ______________

Father's Name: ____

Occupation: ____

Work Phone: ( ) ____________________ Home Phone: ( ) ______________

Religion: ______________ School grade completed: ________ Sex: Male or Female (*circle one*)

Birthdate: ______/______/______ Age when camp opens: _____ Age at onset of diabetes:_____

Full name of camper's primary care physician: ______________________________

Physician's Address: ____

City: ______________________ State: ______ Zip: ________ Phone#: ( ) __________

Diabetes health care provider (if other than above): ______________________________

Address: ____

City: ______________________ State: ______ Zip: ________ Phone#: ( ) __________

Does child usually give own insulin injections? ______________________________

Reactions: Never ___ Occasional ___ Frequent ___ Reactions mild? ___ Severe? ___

Camper Application Form (*continued*) **Form A1**

Camper's Name: ______________________________

Ever lose consciousness?______ Hypoglycemic seizures? ______

Does child recognize signs of own insulin reactions? Yes or No (*circle one*).

What are the usual symptoms of a reaction in your child?

____

____

____

What is used to treat the reactions? ______________________________

How often does child go to bathroom at night? __________________

Bedwetting: Yes or No (*circle one*) Often: Yes or No (*circle one*)

Method of blood sugar testing at home: ______________________________

How often: __________ By whom: ______________________________

Method of urine testing at home:______________________________

How often: __________ By whom: ______________________________

QUESTION	**ANSWER** (*circle one*)	**ADDITIONAL INFORMATION**
Has child ever been in diabetic ketoacidosis?	Yes No	Last episode? __________
Is child subject to frequent colds?	Yes No	
Sore Throat?	Yes No	
Hives/Skin Disease?	Yes No	
Poison Ivy?	Yes No	
Athletes Foot?	Yes No	Date of last physical exam: _____/_____/_____.
Has this person menstruated?	Yes No	
Has she been told about it?	Yes No	
Surgeries?	Yes No	
Allergies	Yes No	List: __________

Chronic health problems/disabilities? ______________________________

____

From what source did you first learn about this camp? ______________________________

List all medications other than insulin (dosage & frequency). **Form A2**

Medication: ____________________
Dosage: ____________________
Frequency: ____________________
Medication: ____________________
Dosage: ____________________
Frequency: ____________________

Medication: ____________________
Dosage: ____________________
Frequency: ____________________
Medication: ____________________
Dosage: ____________________
Frequency: ____________________

Medication: ____________________
Dosage: ____________________
Frequency: ____________________
Medication: ____________________
Dosage: ____________________
Frequency: ____________________

Medication: ____________________
Dosage: ____________________
Frequency: ____________________
Medication: ____________________
Dosage: ____________________
Frequency: ____________________

Form A3

Prospective Campers Application

PLEASE ATTACH BELOW:

CURRENT IMMUNIZATION CERTIFICATE

(Place Here)

PROSPECTIVE CAMPER **Form B**

CAMPER INFORMATION FORM

To be completed by Parent or Legal Guardian

Dear Parent:

The counselor and program staff would like to become acquainted with the camper before camp begins. Please complete the questions below.

Camper's Full Name: ______________________________

Name or nickname camper goes by: ______________________________

Camper's Age: __________ School grade completed: ______________________________

Will this be camper's first time to attend diabetes camp? Yes or No (*circle one*)

If no, please list name and date of other camps attended:

NAME OF CAMP	DATES

Is this camper's first time away from home? Yes No (*circle one*)

Is camper excited about coming to camp? Yes No (*circle one*) If not, why is he/she reluctant?

____

____

WHAT DOES CAMPER ENJOY DOING?	ANY SPECIAL SKILLS OR INTERESTS?

Can camper swim? Yes No Does camper make friends easily? Yes No

Does camper participate in his/her diabetes care? If so, what does he/she do?

____

What new diabetes skills would camper like to learn at camp?

____

____

As a parent, do you have any special concerns or comments?

____

____

Camper Information Form (*continued*) **Form B**

Behavior: Appropriate ______ Hyperactive______ Withdrawn______ Aggressive______

	NEVER	SOMETIMES	MOST ALWAYS
Gets angry when he/she does not get own way	____	____	____
Yells or Screams	____	____	____
Fidgets (cannot sit still)	____	____	____
Touches objects after being told not to	____	____	____
Hits adults	____	____	____
Purposely tries to annoy adults	____	____	____
Repeats misbehavior after being told not to	____	____	____
Uses a particular movement or sound repeatedly	____	____	____
Urinates in places other than the toilet	____	____	____
Bangs objects together	____	____	____
Puts things in mouth	____	____	____
Destroys toys or other objects	____	____	____
Annoys other children	____	____	____
Bites or kicks other children	____	____	____
Runs away (i.e., in stores, on playground)	____	____	____
Acts fearful or anxious	____	____	____

What behavior management techniques work best for you with your child?

____

____

What does your child do well? ____

____

Does your child seem to enjoy interacting with peers? Yes No (*circle one*)

How does your child relate to groups? ____________________________________

____

How does your child relate with one or two peers? ___________________________

____

Has your child been a member of other group activities? Yes No (*circle one*)

Please List:

____________________ ____________________ ____________________

Please summarize the personal care/supervision you feel your child will need at camp (beside routine diabetes management) ____

____

PROSPECTIVE CAMPER **Form C**

CONSENT FORM

I hereby apply for admission of my child (name) ______________________________
to the summer camp for children with diabetes operated by the American Diabetes Association and I understand my child will be subject to the same camp rules as other children. I consent to my child being given the diet, insulin dosage and daily blood glucose monitoring as deemed best by the physician in charge and to my child being given other medical care and testing that may be medically necessary while my child is a camp resident, including tuberculin test and x-ray if test is positive, and including blood testing for Hepatitis B and/or HIV antibodies, in case of accidental finger prick with possibly contaminated material (such as a syringe needle or lancet). I further consent to the release of any test results to the Public Health Authorities, if such release is required by any law, statute, or regulation. I also consent to my child being photographed and that any such photographs may be used for publicity, fund raising or other purposes as determined by the American Diabetes Association, (insert name) Area Office. My child has my permission to leave the campsite on occasional trips to nearby points of interest under the supervision of the Camp Staff.

I understand that while the ADA will supply insulin, syringes, monitoring supplies and routine first aid care required at camp, I shall be responsible for the cost of all other medical treatment of my child, including but not limited to laboratory test, x-rays, and emergency treatment at a hospital or clinic.
In order to assist in the prompt treatment of my child, I hereby consent to any necessary medical or surgical treatment and testing of my child of an emergency nature. Below my signature, I have listed the policy number for any applicable policies of hospitalization insurance which I carry on this child (including Medical Assistance).

I authorize the appropriate representative of the ADA to release the information concerning my hospitalization insurance to any provider of medical or surgical services to my child.
In consideration of the ADA allowing my child to attend its summer camp, I hereby release the ADA, its agents, employees, assigns, volunteers and medical staff, from any and all liability arising out of and in connection with my child's participation in camp for any reason other than the negligence of the American Diabetes Association.

Signature of Parent or Legal Guardian

______________________	______________________	__________
Father	Mother	Date

Insurance Company ______________________________________

Policy Number ____________________ Group Number ____________________

Name of Policy Holder ______________________________________

PROSPECTIVE CAMPER **Form D**

CAMPER DIET FORM

Please be sure to complete all appropriate sections of this form. This will ensure that all campers are given adequate food while at camp. It is also important that accurate information is given. Please do not list what your prescribed meal plan is unless that is what you follow at least 3/4 of the time. We want to know what you are actually eating.

Camper's Name: ______________________________ Age: _____

Height: _________ Weight: _________ Sex: Male ____ Female _____

Name of Parent/Guardian: ______________________________

Address: ______________________________
(Street)

____
(City) (State) (Zip)

Does the camper have any special dietary needs?

____

Food Allergies? ______________ Food Avoidances? ______________

Eating Disorders: ______________ Total Daily Calories (if known): ______________

Please list on the next page two examples of foods and amounts for meals/snacks that might be eaten by the camper. (If the camper is over 12 years old, please allow them to complete this section).

Camper Diet Form (*continued*) **Form D**

Breakfast Example 1 ____________________

Example 2 ____________________

Morning Snack Example 1 ____________________

Example 2 ____________________

Lunch Example 1 ____________________

Example 2 ____________________

Afternoon Snack Example 1 ____________________

Example 2 ____________________

Evening Meal Example 1 ____________________

Example 2 ____________________

Bedtime Snack Example 1 ____________________

Example 2 ____________________

Usual Meal Plan at Home—*please check one:*

_____No Concentrated Sweets _____ Carbohydrate Counting

Please record pattern: ____________________

____

____

Exchange Pattern: Specify number of Calories ____________

Please record pattern: ____________________

____

____

We will use the examples given to devise a meal plan for your camper; please be sure this information is as close to usual as possible.

While at camp, diets may be altered to accommodate the increased energy needs often required because of more vigorous activity. Be assured that Registered Dietitians who work often with children and adolescents with diabetes will be making any changes that are necessary.

PROSPECTIVE CAMPER **Form E**

CAMPER/PARENT AGREEMENT ON CAMP RULES

I will not leave the property for any reason during the camping session.

I will not intentionally injure or endanger myself or any other person either physically or emotionally. This includes keeping my blood sugar extremely high or low on purpose.

I will not destroy/endanger the environment, camp or property of camp or personal property of others. If I do my family will be liable for damages caused.

I will not use foul or abusive language.

I will not engage in any sexual contact.

I will not smoke, use drugs, alcohol, or weapons.

Proximity. If I am with someone who is breaking one of the above rules, I will also be dismissed. If I do not follow these rules, I

1) Will be promptly dismissed from camp.
2) Must have parent/guardian come to camp to pick me up.
3) Will not be refunded camp fees.
4) Risk losing the privilege of returning to camp in the future.

I have read and understand the rules and will help enforce them. In addition, I have read and explained the camp rules to my child and believe that he/she understands them. I agree to pick my child up from camp if this contract is broken by him/her.

____________________________ ____________________________

Camper Signature Parent/Guardian Signature

Date ________________ Date ________________

PROSPECTIVE CAMPER

Form F

HEALTH HISTORY FORM

To be filled out by camper's diabetes health care provider

Dear Doctor:

Your cooperation in supplying the following information about an applicant for (insert camp name) will be greatly appreciated. **The child will not be accepted at camp without this form.**

Name of applicant: ______________________ Sex: (circle one) M F

Date of Birth: ___/___/___ Age at onset of diabetes: ______ Height ______ Weight ______

Last hemoglobin A1C: __________(normal range __________) Date: ______________

Blood glucose range: Pre-breakfast __________ Pre-lunch__________

Pre-supper__________ Bedtime __________

What is child's nutrition program? ______________________

Please Note: It may be necessary, with more exercise to increase caloric intake. This will be done under the camp physician's supervision and noted in the camper's chart.

INDICATE THE INSULIN DOSE LAST PRESCRIBED FOR THE CHILD

UNITS/TYPE	**UNITS/TYPE**
Before Breakfast__________	Before Lunch __________
Before Supper __________	Before Bedtime __________

PLEASE CIRCLE ALL THAT APPLY

Lilly (Humulin)		N, L, U, R, 70/30, 50/50, Humalog
Novo-Nordisk (Novolin)		N, L, R, 70/30
Other (Specify)__________		
Pen	Pump	Velosulin

Note: If insulin dose is changed during camp parent will be notified at departure interview.

Have any complications of diabetes or disabilities been detected? Yes No (*circle one*)

If yes, please specify:______________________

Date of last ophthalmology exam (if known) ______________________

Comments: ______________________

____

Physician's name (typed or printed)______________________

Address: ______________________

______________________ Phone: ( ) ______________

Physician's Signature: ______________________

Mail Form To:

APPENDIX C

Scholarship Application

Please complete and return by ____/____/____

Dear Parents:

In order for your child to be considered for a scholarship for Camp _______, the Camp Committee would like you to complete the following form. No scholarship can be awarded without this form on file. The information will be strictly confidential.

This form should be completed and returned to the ________________ ADA Area Office AS SOON AS POSSIBLE! You will be notified by mail of the scholarship award in late May. Please list all circumstances that may be affecting your need for a scholarship. If you need more space, please attach a separate sheet of paper.

If you have questions regarding this form, please contact ____________________________________.

PLEASE PRINT OR TYPE

Campers Name:______________________________ Age: ________

Father's Name:____________________________ Living:_____ Deceased:_____

Father's Address: ______________________________________

____

(City) (State) (Zip)

Father's Phone(______) ________________

Mother's Name:____________________________ Living:_____ Deceased:_____

Mother's Address: ______________________________________

____

(City) (State) (Zip)

Mother's Phone(______) ________________

Total number of people living in household : ______ Children: ______ Ages: __________

Sources of income: (Please provide sources of income for both mother and father if possible)

Place of Employment: ______________________ Occupation: ______________

Place of Employment: ______________________ Occupation: ______________

Please list below any other sources of income:

AFDC	$__________	Alimony/Child Support	$__________
Food Stamps	$__________	Insurance Dividends	$__________
Pension	$__________	Social Security	$__________
Welfare	$__________	Veterans Benefits	$__________
Disability	$__________	Other ________	$__________

TOTAL Household Income: $____________ (ALL SOURCES)

Does your child receive free or reduced lunch at school? Yes_____ No _____

Does you child attend public school? Yes_____ No _____

Monthly Expenditures:

Housing Pmt	$__________	Insurance	$__________
Utilities Cost	$__________	Medical Expense	$__________
Food Costs	$__________	Auto Expense	$__________

Other monthly expenses: ____________________________________

____

Other reasons for needing a scholarship ____________________________

____

Additional comments ____

____

____

____

Amount you will pay in addition to the deposit: $______________

Is this your first time applying for a scholarship? Yes_____ No _____

If no, when did you apply? (please give year) ____________

How much were you awarded? $__________________

Parent/Guardian Signature ___________________________ Date __________

APPENDIX D

Hypoglycemia & Hyperglycemia

Warning Signs

Photocopy the following pages and give it to anyone who will be watching over your child at camp.

Low Blood Sugar (Hypoglycemia)

Hypoglycemia occurs when blood sugar levels are too low. Many things can cause this, including:

- too much insulin or not enough food
- missed meals or snacks
- more exercise than usual

At camp, all of these are distinct possibilities. Though most children at camp are old enough to recognize the symptoms on their own, it's important to look for warning signs. If a child's blood sugar gets low enough, it's hard for them to think rationally and they may not be able to tell you there's something wrong.

Mild to Moderate Symptoms

Shakiness, trembling	Pale skin
Sweating	Rapid pulse
Hunger	Irritability, crying

Poor coordination	Dizziness
Fatigue, sleepiness	Headache
Slurred speech	Lack of concentration, daydreaming

What to do

- ▲ Do not leave child unattended
- ▲ Test blood sugar
- ▲ Give carbohydrate food or beverage (e.g., non-diet soda, fruit juice, sugar cubes, hard candy)
- ▲ Check blood sugar level after 15 minutes
- ▲ Give some more carbohydrate if blood sugar level is still <80
- ▲ When the child feels better, feed a meal or snack as soon as possible
- ▲ If no meal or snack is scheduled, give crackers with cheese or peanut butter, half a sandwich, or a bowl of cereal with milk
- ▲ Give child time to recover

Severe Symptoms

Loss of consciousness
Seizures

What to do

- ▲ Have the camp nurse, or designated person, give the child a glucagon injection immediately and call for emergency medical assistance
- ▲ Notify child's parents and physician immediately

High Blood Sugar (Hyperglycemia)

Hyperglycemia occurs when the blood sugar gets too high, which usually happens when:

- ▲ the body gets too little insulin, too much food, or not enough exercise
- ▲ the body is under stress from illness

Symptoms

Excessive thirst
Fatigue, weakness
Increase in trips to the bathroom
Blurred vision

What to do

- Check blood sugar level
- Give sugar-free beverages
- Make sure they get to the camp nurse

Index

About the American Diabetes Association

The American Diabetes Association is the nation's leading voluntary health organization supporting diabetes research, information, and advocacy. Its mission is to prevent and cure diabetes and to improve the lives of all people affected by diabetes. The American Diabetes Association is the leading publisher of comprehensive diabetes information. Its huge library of practical and authoritative books for people with diabetes covers every aspect of self-care—cooking and nutrition, fitness, weight control, medications, complications, emotional issues, and general self-care.

To order American Diabetes Association books: Call 1-800-232-6733. http://store.diabetes.org [Note: there is no need to use **www** when typing this particular Web address]

To join the American Diabetes Association: Call 1-800-806-7801. www.diabetes.org/membership

For more information about diabetes or ADA programs and services: Call 1-800-342-2383. E-mail: Customerservice@diabetes.org www.diabetes.org

To locate an ADA/NCQA Recognized Provider of quality diabetes care in your area: Call 1-703-549-1500 ext. 2202. www.diabetes.org/recognition/Physicians/ListAll.asp

To find an ADA Recognized Education Program in your area: Call 1-888-232-0822. www.diabetes.org/recognition/education.asp

To join the fight to increase funding for diabetes research, end discrimination, and improve insurance coverage: Call 1-800-342-2383. www.diabetes.org/advocacy

To find out how you can get involved with the programs in your community: Call 1-800-342-2383. See below for program Web addresses.

American Diabetes Month: Educational activities aimed at those diagnosed with diabetes—month of November. www.diabetes.org/ADM
American Diabetes Alert: Annual public awareness campaign to find the undiagnosed—held the fourth Tuesday in March. www.diabetes.org/alert
The Diabetes Assistance & Resources Program (DAR): diabetes awareness program targeted to the Latino community. www.diabetes.org/DAR
African American Program: diabetes awareness program targeted to the African American community. www.diabetes.org/africanamerican
Awakening the Spirit: Pathways to Diabetes Prevention & Control: diabetes awareness program targeted to the Native American community. www.diabetes.org/awakening

To find out about an important research project regarding type 2 diabetes: www.diabetes.org/ada/research.asp

To obtain information on making a planned gift or charitable bequest: Call 1-888-700-7029. www.diabetes.org/ada/plan.asp

To make a donation or memorial contribution: Call 1-800-342-2383. www.diabetes.org/ada/cont.asp